AF553401

Women's Work, Health and Empowerment

WOMEN'S WORK, HEALTH AND EMPOWERMENT

Anjali Gandhi

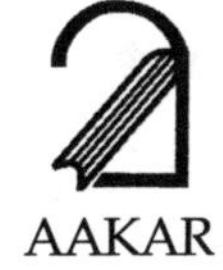

AAKAR

This book is the result of recommendations of the Seminar on
''National Policy of Empowerment of Women''
jointly organized by Sarojini Naidu Centre for
Women's Studies and the Department of Social Work,
Jamia Millia Islamia, New Delhi

WOMEN'S WORK, HEALTH AND EMPOWERMENT

First Published, 2006

ISBN 81-87879-71-8 (Hb)

Published by
AAKAR BOOKS
28 E Pocket IV, Mayur Vihar Phase I, Delhi-110 091
Phone : 011-2279 5505 Telefax : 011-2279 5641
E-mail : aakarb@del2.vsnl.net.in

Printed at
Arpit Printographers, Shahdara Delhi–110 032

Contents

Contributors

Adarsh Sharma, Former Director, NIPCCD, New Delhi

Anjali Gandhi, Professor, Department of Social Work and Honorary Director, Sarojini Naidu Centre for Women's Studies, Jamia Millia Islamia, New Delhi

Ashwani Kumar, Director, Santulan, New Delhi

Kamla Sankaran, Reader, Faculty of Law, University of Delhi, Delhi

K.K. Singh, Additional Director, NIPCCD, New Delhi

Hajira Kumar, Professor and Head, Department of Social Work, Jamia Millia Islamia, New Delhi

Harvinder Kaur, Programme Coordinator, Travellers Aid, Atlanta, U.S.A.

Manisha Sethi, Assistant Editor, Biblio : A Review of Books, New Delhi

Neeti Malhotra, Deputy Head, Governance and Social Justice Unit, British Council, New Delhi

Paul Sachdev, Professor, School of Social Work, Memorial University, New Foundland, Canada

Susheela Kaushik, Former Director, Women's Studies Development Centre, University of Delhi, Delhi

Sushma Batra, Professor, Department of Social Work, University of Delhi, Delhi

Zubair Meenai, Reader, Department of Social Work, Jamia Millia Islamia, New Delhi

Introduction

World over, status differences are based on the universal dimensions of age and gender. Whereas sex is a biological concept, gender is a social construct which specifies the socially and culturally prescribed roles that men and women are supposed to follow. In her book *The Creation of Patriarchy*, Gerda Lerner describes gender as "the costume, a mask, a straitjacket in which men and women dance their unequal dance". Gender is thus a product of human thought and culture. Consequently gender differs between societies and across the social, ethnic and cultural groups within societies. So pervasive is the influence of gender that it permeates every aspect of a person's life and determines the roles, responsibilities, aspirations, and even choice of work/career. Gender discrimination is recognized by many as the worst form of subordination which has resulted in the denial of necessities, opportunities, and aspirations for women.

The Convention on Elimination of all Forms of Discrimination Against Women (CEDAW) adopted in 1979 by the UN General Assembly, defines what constitutes discrimination against women and sets up an agenda for national action to end such discrimination. State parties who have signed the Convention have agreed to take all appropriate measures, including legislation and temporary special measures, so that women can enjoy all their human rights and fundamental freedoms. As of March 2005, 180 countries — over ninety per cent of the members of the United Nations — are party to the Convention, binding themselves to do nothing in contravention of its terms. India is also a signatory to the Convention.

The Fourth World Conference on Women in Beijing in 1995 and now the Beijing +5 initiatives (specifically the twenty third special session of the General Assembly on Women 2000: Gender Equality, Development and Peace for the Twenty First Century) reaffirmed the importance of gender mainstreaming in all areas and at all levels and the complementarity between mainstreaming and special activities targeting women. Certain areas were identified as requiring focussed attention. These included: education; social services and health (including sexual and reproductive health); the HIV/AIDS pandemic; violence against women and girls; the persistent and increasing burden of poverty on women; vulnerability of migrant women including exploitation and trafficking; natural disaster and environmental management; the development of strong, effective and accessible national machineries for the advancement of women; and the formulation of strategies to enable women and men to reconcile and share work and family responsibilities equally. In addition to this the General Assembly, while adopting the recommendations of this special session in the year 2005, reaffirmed the need for the mobilisation of resources at the national and international levels, the promotion of an active and visible policy of mainstreaming a gender perspective by the United Nations, including through the work of the Special Advisor on Gender Issues and Advancement of Women and through the maintenance of gender units and focal points.

In response to this imperative laid down by the United Nations, the Government of India has adopted a National Policy for Empowerment of Women in 2001. Equal stress is being laid down on the widespread dissemination of this policy particularly amongst stakeholders. One such initiative for the dissemination and discussion on the policy was taken by the Sarojini Naidu Centre for Women's Studies and the Department of Social Work, Jamia Millia Islamia through a Seminar on the National Policy for Empowerment of Women. More than 100 academicians, NGO workers, policy makers and civil servants participated in a two-day Seminar on 7–8 March 2002. The seminar was organized with the support of the Department of Women and Child Development, Government of India.

One of the key agreements between the participants of the seminar was that adequate resource material should be developed on a variety of women's issues so that more effective work on women's issues can be done. As a result, this publication was initiated. The end product is by no means comprehensive since women's lives are affected by a plethora of issues. In this publication, an attempt has been made to present a few issues related to women ranging from work, religion, HIV/AIDS to mental health and leprosy.

Given the focus on India's National Policy for women in the seminar, it is pertinent to begin with **K.K. Singh**'s paper on women empowerment in relation to the national policy, for it traces the national and international efforts to ensure equality of opportunity and empowerment of women. India signed and ratified the Convention on Elimination of all Forms of Discrimination Against Women (CEDAW) in 1993. Despite efforts, the author notes that gender disparity remains and social stereotyping and violence at domestic and societal levels continue. The attempts of the National Policy for Empowerment of Women (2001) are then enumerated in detail.

Research shows that women and girls tend to work harder than men, are more likely to invest their earnings in their children, are major producers as well as consumers and shoulder critical, life-sustaining responsibilities without which men and boys could not survive, much less enjoy high levels of productivity.

Kamala Sankaran in her paper on women, work and empowerment explains similar issues. There are more women than men work in the unorganized sector. The effect of casualization has pushed more women into the unorganized sector. Women workers thus must be encouraged to join organizations that defend their interests. Patriarchal norms have relegated women's work performed at home as unimportant or being for self-consumption by family members. Only after the 1991 census, activities for self-consumption and unpaid work for family enterprises were also considered to be work. But even this leaves out unpaid domestic work performed by women. Largely, women's position in the labour market is worse than that of men with work performed by women being undervalued and low paid.

Research from around the world has also shown that 'gender down' inequality tends to slow economic growth and make the rise from poverty more difficult. The reasons for this are not hard to understand. Half of the world's population is female, hence the extent to which women and girls benefit from development policies and programmes has a major impact on countries' overall development success. That is the reason that the third Millennium Development Goal — to promote gender equality and empower women — is a central component of the World Bank's mission to reduce poverty and stimulate economic growth. Women's access to micro finance has proved to be quite successful.

Discussing women's empowerment through micro-credit, **Zubair Meenai** opens his paper by citing evidence from the world over about how gender inequalities undermine the effectiveness of development policies. In terms of work, for instance, work done by women is largely undervalued and unrecognised and they continue to earn lower wages for the same work as compared to men. Women continue to have a systematically poorer command over a range of products, resources including land, information and financial resources. In response to women's expressed need for improved access to credit, particularly to small loans which allow them to engage in risk averse, multi production strategies and thereby to improve the livelihoods of their families, thrift and credit or self-help groups have been promoted both by the government and the NGOs. The author points out how, with the introduction of micro-finance in the eighties, by the late nineties there was a substantial body of evidence to show that micro credit was indeed a compelling anti-poverty and development strategy. The paper then offers divergent views of scholars over the effectiveness of micro-credit in the economic empowerment of women. It also shows that credit for empowerment extends beyond its prima facie objective of providing access to credit only. It creates community-owned institutions as well where women are empowered when savings, credit and enterprise are used as tools for mobilizing and building capacities of grassroot women collectives.

Adequate resource allocation and optional spending can bring about an incremental change in the lives of women. This need has been recognized for some time now, with the 23rd special session of UN General Assembly urging all nations to integrate a gender perspective into key macroeconomic and social development policies. Tracing the history of gender budgeting in her paper 'Gender Budgeting and Auditing : Insights from the Indian Experiences', **Adarsh Sharma** clarifies that gendering the budget is not a means to bargain for a larger share of the resources for women or create a separate budget for them. The aim is to analyse the budgetary expenditures from a gender perspective.

Amongst the many provisions highlighted in the National Policy is that of ensuring elimination of discrimination against women in the political and public life of the country. These are noble aspirations, as **Susheela Kaushik** points out in her paper on 'Women in Governance in India', but the ground reality is that women representation in decision-making position is negligible. Notwithstanding the guarantee in India towards political equality, women's participation in the voting progress has always been less than that of males ever since the first general election in 1952. The author notes that although women's participation in governance and policy-making level is low, their participation has become considerably visible at the local government level in rural and urban areas. Describing the women-focussed agendas of political parties, the challenges and obstacles women face in getting a better share and the persistent gaps that exist between intention and implementation, the author concludes that education and skills-building of women will go a long way in providing them equal opportunities in governance.

Religion, through its doctrines and strictures, plays a significant role in the lives of women. Since India is a land of many religions, an attempt has been made in this publication to present an analytical view of impact of Jainism and Islam on the lives of women.

Hajira Kumar in her situational analysis on 'Education among Muslim Women' cites evidence from Islamic scriptures to show how Islam favours learning. Women of early Islamic days, she notes, excelled in religious teaching, medicine, nursing, trade and social service. However, contemporary Indian Muslim women are segregated, disempowered, and marginalised. This leads to low self-esteem, the author points out.

Exploring how stated ideologies of religion differ from lived realities, **Manisha Sethi**'s paper focuses on the status of Jain women in India. Commenting on the irony of the fact that Jainism emerged as a challenge to orthodox Brahminical practices and offered a more equal status to women, she discovers that reality is quite the contrary. Citing some relevant cases, the paper traces how, by the time the Indian Constitution was adopted, Jains were said to be included amongst 'Hindus' as per Article 25. Therefore, with respect to personal laws the validity of a separate legal code as having an impact on say, rights of inheritance was rejected. Another aspect that the paper elucidates is the participation of a large number of Jain women in its ascetic orders. Jain *sadhvis* (i.e. women ascetics) are in fact central to the perpetuation of their community and religious life. The paper also points at the contradiction in Jain texts where on the one hand, a woman is hailed for her spiritual achievements and on the other, condemned for being an 'evil temptress'. Even in the religious order, a gendered hierarchy remains as nuns are expected to show deference to monks. Some instances of women ascetics protesting against this have been reported. But spiritual opportunities provided to women have not resulted in social empowerment.

Closely linked to the issues of employment are the post-retirement changes that are unique to women. **Sushma Batra,** in her paper on retired women, studies the changing social roles of women upon retirement. One hundred and fifty women in the age group of 60–70 years were interviewed after they had retired as school teachers, public servants or professionals. The paper studies how their life is affected after retirement, what their continuing or new roles are after retirement and which roles have terminated. It was found that the roles most likely affected after retirement are health status, gainful utilization of time and network relationship. On the other hand, not much change was seen in their family life, living arrangements and financial status. The paper concludes that loss of power and absence of decision-making in their lives made more women feel that they had 'no role' to play.

Due to the caring and nurturing role that women perform, they largely tend to neglect their health. Resources are generally spent on a more wholesome diet and quick treatment for the male members of the family. And in the case of stigma-related diseases such as HIV/AIDS and leprosy, the delay and also denial of treatment becomes even more common for women.

HIV/AIDS is also a gendered disease. Not only are women biologically at a higher risk of getting infected with HIV as compared to men, the impact of HIV is more severe for women due to the social, legal, familial and personal ramifications. **Neeti Malhotra,** in her paper on gender issues in HIV/AIDS, discusses how the dominant world view of women being subservient to men has also translated into HIV/AIDS prevention programmes where women are largely seen as carriers or vectors of the disease. Gender-sensitive and gender-transformative interventions are needed to make for effective strategies in preventing HIV/AIDS. Training of personnel particularly social workers is very important for preventing AIDS since it poses a formidable challenge for them in terms of what can be done on behalf of clients and also how to respond professionally. **Paul Sachdev** conducted a study of 385 second-year graduate social work students enrolled in eleven colleges of four states— Maharashtra, Karnataka (high HIV/AIDS prevalence states), Delhi and Haryana which have low to medium incidence of HIV/AIDS.

The study underscores the need for more in-depth and comprehensive presentation of HIV/AIDS specific knowledge as well as affective exploration of attitudes. The author stresses that the importance of the acceptance of and commitment to gender equality, especially among male students should be of high priority when disseminating educational content. Training strategies, Professor Sachdev recommends, must focus on social skills based on learning and cognitive behavioural theory to implement behaviour change. His study also highlights the need for assessment of the HIV/AIDS curricula to gauge their effectiveness.

Another health issue which is gaining concern and ground the world over for the sheer impact it is going to have is that of mental health. **Ashwani Kumar**'s paper on gender and mental health provides evidence from research to show that women are disproportionately affected by mental health disorders. Symptoms of depression and anxiety as well as psychiatric disorders and psychological distress are more common among women. Gender differences in psychiatric morbidity in most parts of the world are explained by poverty, isolation, violence, problems related to parenting and child care which affect women more. The author contends that, while gender mainstreaming in addressing mental health issues is important, 'healthy' policies aimed at improving the social status of women are needed along with 'health' policies targeting the entire spectrum of women's health needs.

Due to fear of spreading infection, women are either abandoned by their own family members or they choose self-inflicted seclusion. The study by **Harvinder Kaur** on social hurdles in the utilisation of health care facilities by women leprosy patients was conducted on 160 women leprosy patients above 15 years of age, seeking treatment from four hospitals in Delhi—two government and two private-run. The study shows that the women leprosy patients do not reach out for medical help as soon as they notice the symptoms. Due to household responsibilities they tend to ignore their health. Their dependency on others to be escorted was also found to be responsible for their extended treatment gap and treatment compliance. They delay treatment till their symptoms become too grave to bear and disrupt their normal functioning. The social stigma attached to leprosy and dependency on their male counterparts act as treatment hurdles. The author recommends that in the light of low use of treatment facilities by women leprosy patients, among other things, women should be provided education and training in leadership to enhance their sense of self-worth, improve their self-esteem and their right to good health.

As has been stated before, this compilation of articles is by no means complete nor an exhaustive overview of issues confronted by women. These present some of the issues that emerged during deliberations at the Seminar on National Policy on Empowerment of Women held at Jamia Millia Islamia in March 2002 a report of which is given at the end.

More such attempts at studying and compiling views, experiences and learning on issues concerning women's needs should be made on an ongoing basis.

—Anjali Gandhi

Chapter 1

Women Empowerment in Relation to the National Policy for the Empowerment of Women

K.K. Singh

Policy documents concerning Indian women have been guided by the Constitution. The Preamble to the Constitution of India assures "to secure to all its citizens: Justice, social, economic and political; Liberty of thought, expression, belief, faith and worship; Equality of status and opportunity; and to promote among them all Fraternity assuring the dignity of the individual and the unity of the Nation." To attain these national objectives, the Constitution guarantees certain fundamental rights and freedom such as freedom of speech, protection of life, personal liberty and the prohibition of discrimination or denial of equal protection.

Indian women are the beneficiaries of these rights to the same magnitude as Indian men. For instance, Article 14 ensures 'equality before law' and Article 15 'prohibits any discrimination'. There is only one specific provision in Article 15(3), which empowers the State to make 'any special provision for women and children'. This is in violation of the fundamental obligation of non-discrimination among citizens, inter alia, on

---

I thankfully acknowledge the valuable contribution and support extended by my colleague Shri B.R. Siwal, Faculty Member, in preparation of this paper.

the ground of sex. Consequently, this provision has enabled the State to make special provision for women, particularly in the field of labour legislation like the Factories Act, the Mines Act, Child Labour Prohibition (Regulation) Act and so forth. Article 16 (1) guarantees "equality of opportunity for all citizens in matters relating to employment or appointment to any office under the State". And Article 16 (2) forbids discrimination "in respect of any employment of office under the State" on the grounds only of "religion, race, caste, sex, descent, place of birth, residence or any one of them".

Enunciated in Part IV of the Constitution, the Directive Principles of State Policy embody the major policy goals of a welfare state. Together with the chapter on Fundamental Rights, they concretise the Constitutional vision of a new Indian socio-political order. Even though the state is charged with "a duty . . . to apply these principles in making laws" which are ". . . fundamental in the governance of the country" (Article 37), these Principles are declared as non-justifiable. They were made non-enforceable in courts because it was felt that their fulfilment would require a time-dimension of a few decades, whereas the Constitutional values embodied in the Fundamental Rights chapter needed immediate implementation. In the case of the Directive Principles this was not possible save at the cost of the viability of the state.

Juridically, the Directive Principles are a vital part of Indian Constitutional law. Like the Preamble, they reflect high ideals of a liberal democratic polity. They are meant to be used by all agencies of the state as guidelines to action as major goals of policy. Courts can use them as a body of values and standards relevant to the act of judicial choice-making. But the Directive Principles neither confer power nor legislative competence, or give rise to a cause of action for which remedy is available in a court of law, bestow rights, or create remedies. At the same time, they cannot be amended, save through the prescribed procedure. Some of the Directive Principles are "women-specific". Others concern women indirectly or by implication. Amongst those which concern women directly and have a special bearing on their status are: Article 39 (a)—

the right to an adequate means of livelihood for men and women equally; Article 39 (d)—equal pay for equal work for both men and women; Article 39 (e)—protection of the health and strength of workers—men, women and children from abuse and entry into a vocations unsuited to their age and strength; and Article 42— just and humane conditions of work and maternity relief.

In the second category falls the omnibus provision of Article 38 which briefly directs the State to secure a just social, political and economic order, geared to promote the welfare of the people; Article 39 (b), (c) and (f) focus on distribution, ownership and control of material resources of the community for the common good, prevention of concentration of wealth and means of production to the common detriment, and protection of childhood and youth against exploitation, and moral and material abandonment; Article 40—organization of village panchayats to promote self-government; Article 41—right to work, education and public assistance in cases of unemployment, old age, sickness, disablement and other types of underserved wants; Article 43—provision of work, a living wage, conditions of work ensuring a decent standard of life and full enjoyment of leisure, of social and cultural opportunities, and the promotion of cottage industries; Article 44—Uniform Civil Code; Article 45—free and compulsory education for all children up to the age of 14; and Article 47—raising the level of nutrition and the standard of living of the people and improvement of public health.

Plan provisions for development of women have been receiving attention of the government right from the very First Plan (1951–56). But, the same has been treated as a subject of 'welfare' and clubbed together with the welfare of the disadvantaged groups like the destitute, the disabled, the aged, etc. The Central Social Welfare Board (CSWB), set up in 1953, acts as an Apex Body at the national level to promote voluntary action at various levels, especially at the grassroots, to take up welfare-related activities for women and children. The Second to Fifth Plans (1956–79) continued to reflect the very same welfare approach, besides giving priority to women's education, and launching measures to improve maternal and child health services, supplementary feeding for children and expectant and nursing mothers.

In 1971, following a resolution of the Ministry of Education and Social Welfare, the Committee on the Status of Women in India (CSWI) was constituted at the instance of the UN General Assembly. The presentation of the CSWI report "Towards Equality" coincided with the celebration of 1975 as International Women's Year. To operationalise the recommendations of CSWI, a Blueprint of Action Points and National Plan of Action for Women, 1976 was formulated by the then Department of Social Welfare, Government of India. This in turn led to the presentation of the Report of the Working Group on Employment for Women, 1978, as well as the Report of the Working Group on Development of Village-Level Organizations of Rural Women 1978. It also formed a part of the Sixth Five-Year Plan exercise. The impact of these reports resulted in a separate chapter on Women and Development 1980-85 in the Sixth Five-Year Plan. It also resulted in women being perceived as productive contributors to the nation's economy.

Following an agreement signed between the then Ministry of Agriculture and Irrigation, Government of India and the Food and Agricultural Organization (UN), a Report of the National Committee on Role and Participation of Women in Agriculture and Rural Development 1980 was submitted. Further, the report of the Working Group on Personnel Policies for Bringing Greater Involvement of Women in Science and Technology—1981 outlined the extent of participation of women in scientific establishments and suggested measures for enhancing involvement of women in science and technology. In the Seventh Five-Year Plan, the chapter on Socio-Economic Programmes for Women—1985–90 moved further away from a 'welfare' approach to a more positive 'developmental' approach to women's concerns. The Indian Parliament also adopted a National Policy on Education—1986 which laid special emphasis on education of women and girls in all fields including science and technology.

The shift in the approach from 'welfare' to 'development' of women could take place only in the Sixth Plan (1980–85). Accordingly, the Sixth Plan adopted a multi-disciplinary approach with a special thrust on the three core sectors of health, education and employment. In the Seventh Plan (1985–90), the developmental programmes continued with the major objective of raising their economic and social status and bringing them into the mainstream of national development. A significant step in this direction was to identify and promote the Beneficiary-Oriented Schemes (BOS) in various developmental sectors which extended direct benefits to women. The thrust on generation of both skilled and unskilled employment through proper education and vocational training continued. The Eighth Plan (1992–97), with human development as its major focus, played a very important role in the development of women. It promised to ensure that benefits of development from different sectors do not bypass women, implement special programmes to complement the general development programmes and to monitor the flow of benefits to women from other development sectors and enable women to function as equal partners and participants in the development process.

The Ninth Plan (1997–2002) made two significant changes in the conceptual strategy of planning for women. Firstly, 'Empowerment of Women' became one of the nine primary objectives of the Plan. To this effect, the Approach of the Plan was to create an enabling environment where women could freely exercise their rights both within and outside home, as equal partners along with men. Secondly, the Plan attempted 'convergence of existing services' available in both women-specific and women-related sectors. With these aims, it directed both the centre and the states to adopt a special strategy of 'Women's Component Plan' (WCP) through which not less than 30 per cent of funds/benefits flow to women from all the general development sectors. It also suggested that a special vigil be kept on the flow of the earmarked funds/ benefits through an effective mechanism to ensure that the proposed strategy brings forth a holistic approach towards empowering women.

In recent years, the empowerment of women has been recognised as the central issue in determining the status of women. The National Commission for Women was set up by an Act of Parliament in 1990 to safeguard the rights and legal entitlements of women. The 73rd and 74th Amendments (1993) to the Constitution of India have provided for reservation of seats in the local bodies of Panchayats and Municipalities for women, laying a strong foundation for their participation in decision-making at the local levels.

In addition to this the Report of the National Expert Committee on Women Prisoners (1987) identified the gaps and drawbacks in existing facilities and services. It recommended a more humane policy for them. The National Commission on Self-Employed Women and Women in the Informal Sector was appointed in January 1987. This was yet another landmark development which looked into the ways and means to ameliorate the suffering of the unprotected labouring women. In its report entitled *Shramshakti* submitted in June 1988, the Commission outlined many comprehensive policy recommendations towards this end. Also in 1987, a Core Group was set up by the Department of Women and Child Development to formulate a National Perspective Plan for Women 1988–2000 A.D. The report was released in October 1988.

INTERNATIONAL EFFORTS

The year 1975 was declared as International Women's Year by the United Nations. As a result of the World Conference held during June–July 1975, promulgated 30 principles on the equality of women and their contribution to national development and international peace. Also, the Action Plan stipulated 14 minimum objectives to be met before the mid-term appraisal in 1980. In December 1979 the UN General Assembly adopted the Convention on the Elimination of All Forms of Discrimination Against Women. At present, India is also a signatory to this convention with some reservation(s).

A mid-term appraisal, Programme of Action for the Second

Half of the United Nations, Decade for Women: Equality, Development and Peace of the World Plan of Action adopted by the World Conference of the International Women's Year, took place in Copenhagen in July 1980. The Ministry of Social Welfare, Government of India prepared a paper, India—A Status Paper—1980 to review India's progress in attaining the minimum objectives. The paper also highlighted the constraints and problems faced in promoting participation of women in development. The United Nations Economic and Social Commission for Asia and the Pacific held a preparatory meeting for the World Conference on Women, at the Ministerial level in March 1984. The deliberations of the meeting resulted in the report of the Regional Intergovernmental Preparatory meeting of the World Conference to Review and Appraise the Achievements of the United Nations Decade for Woman: Equality, Development and Peace—1984. At the ministerial level, another conference took place in April 1985 of the Non-Aligned and other Developing Countries. The intention was to approach the World Conference on Women with full knowledge of their achievements and failures, as well as to evolve a strategy to tackle the problems confronting the world. The recommendations were complied into the New Delhi Document on Women in Development—1985.

At the end of the United Nations Decade for Women, the World Conference was held in Kenya in 1985. The World Conference adopted Forward Looking Strategies for the Advancement of Women—1985 to serve as guidelines for creating a new world order based on equality, development and peace. For the closing conference of the Women' Decade, the Ministry of Social and Women's Welfare, Government of India prepared a document entitled 'Women in India: Country Paper 1985'. This status paper assessed the impact of the decade on the development of women, the constraints that exist and strategies for the advancement of women.

The above description indicates that India has also ratified various international conventions and human rights instruments committing to secure equal rights of women. Key among them is the ratification of the Convention on Elimination of All Forms of Discrimination Against Women (CEDAW) in 1993.

The Mexico Plan of Action (1975), the Nairobi Forward Looking Strategies (1985), the Beijing Declaration as well as the Platform for Action (1995) and the Outcome Document adopted by the UNGA Session on Gender Equality and Development and Peace for the 21st century, titled "Further actions and initiatives to implement the Beijing Declarations and the Platform for Action" have been unreservedly endorsed by India for appropriate follow up. The Policy also takes note of the commitments of the Ninth Five-Year Plan and the other Sectoral Policies relating to Empowerment of Women.

In the field of regional co-operation, the decision was taken in the first summit of the Heads of State or Government of the South Asian Association for Regional Cooperation, 1985. The first Ministerial meeting on Women in Development was held in Shillong in 1986 at the instance of the Government of India. It resulted in publishing the 'Women in Development: Report of SAARC Ministerial Meeting 1986'.

The women's movement and a widespread network of non-government organizations which have strong grassroots presence and deep insight into women's concerns have contributed in inspiring initiatives for the empowerment of women. However, there still exists a wide gap between the goals enunciated in the Constitution, legislation, policies, plans, programmes, and related mechanisms on the one hand and the situational reality of the status of women in India, on the other. This has been analysed extensively in the Report of the Committee on the Status of Women in India: "Towards Equality", 1974 and highlighted in the National Perspective Plan for Women, 1988–2000, the *Shramshakti* Report, 1988 and the "Platform for Action, Five Years After—An Assessment".

Gender disparity manifests itself in various forms, the most obvious being the trend of continuously declining female ratio in the population in the last few decades. Social stereotyping and violence at the domestic and social levels are some of the other manifestations. Discrimination against the girl child, adolescent girls and women persists in parts of the country. The underlying causes of gender inequality are related to social and economic structure, which is based on informal and formal norms, and practices.

Consequently, the access of women, particularly those belonging to weaker sections including Scheduled Castes/ Scheduled Tribes/Other Backward Classes and minorities, majority of whom are in the rural areas and in the informal, unorganised sector—to education, health and productive resources, among others, is inadequate. Therefore, they remain largely marginalised, poor and socially excluded.

NATIONAL POLICY FOR EMPOWERMENT OF WOMEN (2001)

Goal and Objectives

The goal of this Policy is to bring about the advancement, development and empowerment of women. The Policy is widely disseminated so as to encourage active participation of all stakeholders for achieving its goals. Specifically, the objectives of this Policy include:

(i) Creating an environment through positive economic and social policies for full development of women to enable them to realize their full potential.

(ii) The *de jure* and *de facto* enjoyment of all human rights and fundamental freedom by women on equal basis with men in all spheres—political, economic, social, cultural and civil.

(iii) Equal access to participation and decision-making of women in social, political and economic life of the nation.

(iv) Equal access of women to health care, quality education at all levels, career and vocational guidance, employment, equal remuneration, occupational health and safety, social security and public office, etc.

(v) Strengthening legal systems aimed at elimination of all forms of discrimination against women.

(vi) Changing societal attitudes and community practices

by active participation and involvement of both men and women.

(vii) Mainstreaming a gender perspective in the development process.

(viii) Elimination of discrimination and all forms of violence against women and the girl child.

(ix) Building and strengthening partnerships with civil society, particularly women's organizations.

Policy Prescriptions

Judicial Legal Systems

The legal–judicial system is to be made more responsive and gender sensitive to women's needs, especially in cases of domestic violence and personal assault. New laws will be enacted and existing laws reviewed to ensure that justice is quick and the punishment meted out to the culprits is commensurate with the severity of the offence. At the initiative of and with the full participation of all stakeholders including community and religious leaders, the Policy would aim to encourage changes in personal laws such as those related to marriage, divorce, maintenance and guardianship so as to eliminate discrimination against women. The evolution of property rights in a patriarchal system has contributed to the subordinate status of women. The Policy would aim to encourage changes in laws relating to ownership of property and inheritance by evolving consensus in order to make them gender-just.

Decision-Making

Women's equality in power sharing and active participation in decision-making, including decision-making in political process at all levels will be ensured for the achievement of the goals of empowerment. All measures will be taken to guarantee women equal access to and full participation in decision-making bodies at every level, including the legislative, executive, judicial, corporate, statutory bodies, as also the advisory commissions, committees, boards, trusts, etc. Affirmative action such as reservations/quotas, including in higher legislative bodies, will be considered whenever necessary on a time-bound basis. Women-friendly personnel policies will also be drawn up to encourage women to participate effectively in the developmental process.

Mainstreaming a Gender Perspective in the Development Process

Policies, programmes and systems will be established to ensure mainstreaming of women's perspectives in all developmental processes, as catalysts, participants and recipients. Wherever there are gaps in policies and programmes, women-specific interventions would be undertaken to bridge these. Co-ordinating and monitoring mechanisms will also be devised to assess from time to time the progress of such mainstreaming mechanisms. As a result, women's issues and concerns will specially be addressed and reflected in all concerned laws, sectoral policies, plans and programmes of action.

Economic Empowerment of Women

Poverty Eradication

Since women comprise the majority of the population below the poverty line and are very often in situations of extreme poverty, given the harsh realities of intra-household and social discrimination, macro-economic policies and poverty eradication programmes will specifically address the needs and problems of such women. There will be improved implementation of programmes which are already women-oriented with women as special targets. Steps will be taken for mobilisation of poor women and convergence of services, by offering them a range of economic and social options, along with necessary support measures to enhance their capabilities.

Micro Credit

In order to enhance women's access to credit for consumption and production, the establishment of new, and strengthening of existing micro-credit mechanisms and micro-finance institutions will be undertaken so that the outreach of credit is enhanced. Other supportive measures would be taken to ensure adequate flow of credit through extant financial institutions and banks, so that all women below poverty line have easy access to credit.

Women and Economy

Women's perspectives will be included in designing and implementing macro-economic and social policies by institutionalising their participation in such processes. Their contribution to social-economic development as producers and workers will be recognised in the formal and informal sectors (including home-based workers) and appropriate policies relating to employment and to their working conditions will be drawn up. Such measures could include: reinterpretation and redefinition of conventional concepts of work wherever necessary, e.g. in the Census records, to reflect women's contribution as producers and workers.

Globalization

Globalization has presented new challenges for the realization of the goal of women's equality, the gender impact of which has not been systematically evaluated fully. However, from the micro-level studies that were commissioned by the Department of Women and Child Development, it is evident that there is a need for re-framing policies for access to employment and quality of employment. Benefits of the growing global economy have been unevenly distributed leading to wider economic disparities, the feminization of poverty, increased gender inequality through deteriorating working conditions and unsafe working environment especially in the informal economy and rural areas. Strategies will be designed to enhance the capacity of women and empower them to meet the negative social and economic impacts, which may flow from the globalisation process.

Women and Agriculture

In view of the critical role of women in the agriculture and allied sectors, as producers, concerted efforts will be made to ensure that benefits of training, extension and various programmes will reach them in proportion to their numbers. The programmes for training women in soil conservation, social forestry, dairy development and other occupations allied to agriculture like horticulture, livestock including small animal husbandry, poultry, fisheries, etc. will be expanded to benefit women workers in the agriculture sector.

Women and Industry

The important role played by women in electronics, information technology and food processing and agro industry and textiles has been crucial to the development of these sectors. They would be given comprehensive support in terms of labour legislation, social security and other support services to participate in various industrial sectors. Women at present cannot work in night shifts in factories even if they wish to. Suitable measures will be taken to enable women to work in night shifts in factories. This will be accompanied with support services for security, transportation, etc.

Social Empowerment of Women

Education

Equal access to education for women and girls will be ensured. Special measures will be taken to eliminate discrimination, universalise education, eradicate illiteracy, create a gender-sensitive educational system, increase enrolment and retention rates of girls and improve the quality of education to facilitate life-long learning as well as development of occupation/ vocation/technical skills by women. Reducing the gender gap in secondary and higher education would be a focus area. Sectoral time targets in existing policies will be achieved, with special focus on girls and women, particularly those belonging to weaker sections including the Scheduled Castes/Scheduled Tribes/Other Backward Classes/Minorities. Gender-sensitive curricula would be developed at all levels of educational system in order to address sex stereotyping as one of the causes of gender discrimination.

Health

A holistic approach to women's health which includes both nutrition and health services will be adopted and special attention will be given to the needs of women and the girl at all stages of the life cycle. The reduction in infant mortality and maternal mortality, which are sensitive indicators of human development, is a priority concern. This policy reiterates the national demographic goals for Infant Mortality Rate (IMR), Maternal Mortality Rate (MMR) set out in the National Population Policy 2000. Women should have access to comprehensive, affordable and quality health care. Measures will be adopted that take into account the reproductive rights of women to enable them to exercise informed choices, their vulnerability to sexual and health problems together with endemic, infectious and communicable diseases such as malaria, TB, and water-borne diseases as well as hypertension and cardio-pulmonary diseases. The social, developmental and health consequences of HIV/AIDS and other sexually transmitted diseases will be tackled from a gender perspective.

To effectively meet problems of infant and maternal mortality, and early marriage, the availability of proper and accurate data at micro level on deaths, birth and marriages is required. Strict implementation of registration of births and deaths would be ensured and registration of marriages would be made compulsory. In accordance with the commitment of the National Population Policy (2000) to population stabilization, this Policy recognises the critical need of men and women to have access to safe, effective and affordable methods of family planning of their choice and the need to suitably address the issues of early marriages and spacing of children. Interventions such as spread of education, compulsory registration of marriage and special programmes like *Balika Samridhi Yojana* (BSY) should impact on delaying the age of marriage so that by 2010 child marriages are eliminated.

Women's traditional knowledge about health care and nutrition will be recognised through proper documentation and its use will be encouraged. The use of Indian and alternative systems of medicine will be enhanced within the framework of overall health infrastructure available for women.

Nutrition

In view of the high risk of malnutrition and disease that women face at all the three critical states, viz. infancy and childhood, adolescent and reproductive phase, focussed attention would be paid to meeting the nutritional needs of women at all stages of the life cycle. This is also important in view of the critical link between the health of adolescent girls, pregnant and lactating women with the health of infant and young children. Special efforts will be made to tackle the problem of macro and micro nutrient deficiencies especially amongst pregnant and lactating women as it leads to various diseases and disabilities. Intrahousehold discrimination in nutritional matters vis-a-vis girls and women will be sought to be ended through appropriate strategies. Widespread use of nutrition education would be made to address the issues of intra-household imbalances in nutrition and the special needs of pregnant and lactating women. Women's participation will also be ensured in planning, superintendence and delivery of the system.

Drinking Water and Sanitation

Special attention will be given to the needs of women in the provision of safe drinking water, sewage disposal, toilet facilities and sanitation within accessible reach of households, especially in rural areas and urban slums. Women's participation will be ensured in the planning, delivery and maintenance of such services.

Housing and Shelter

Women's perspectives will be included in housing policies, planning of housing colonies and provision of shelter both in rural and urban areas. Special attention will be given for providing adequate housing and accommodation for women including single women, female heads of households, working women, students, apprentices and trainees.

Environment

Women will be involved and their perspectives reflected in the policies and programmes for environment, conservation and restoration. Considering the impact of environmental factors on their livelihood, women's participation will be ensured in the conservation of the environment and control of environmental degradation. The vast majority of rural women still depend on the locally available non-commercial sources of energy such as animal dung, crop waste and fuel wood. In order to ensure the efficient use of these energy resources in an environment-friendly manner, the Policy will aim at promoting the programmes of non-conventional energy resources. Women will be involved in spreading the use of solar energy, biogas, smokeless *chulhas* and other rural application so as to have a visible impact of these measures in influencing eco system and in changing the lifestyles of rural women.

Science and Technology

Programmes will be strengthened to bring about a greater involvement of women in science and technology. These will include measures to motivate girls to take up science and technology for higher education and also ensure that development projects with scientific and technical inputs involve women fully. Efforts to develop a scientific temper and awareness will also be stepped up. Special measures would be taken for their training in areas where they have special skills like communication and information technology. Efforts to develop appropriate technologies suited to women's needs as well as to reduce their drudgery will be given a special focus too.

Women in Difficult Circumstances

In recognition of the diversity of women's situations and in acknowledgement of the needs of specially disadvantaged groups, measures and programmes will be undertaken to provide them with special assistance. These groups include women in extreme poverty, destitute women, women in conflict situations, women affected by natural calamities, women in less developed regions, the disabled widows, elderly women, single women in difficult circumstances, women heading households, those displaced from employment, migrants, women who are victims of marital violence, deserted women and prostitutes, etc.

Violence against women

All forms of violence against women, physical and mental, whether at domestic or societal levels, including those arising from customs, traditions or accepted practices shall be dealt with effectively with a view to eliminate its incidence. Institutions and mechanisms/schemes for assistance will be created and strengthened for prevention of such violence, including sexual harassment at work place and customs like dowry; for the rehabilitation of the victims of violence and for taking effective action against the perpetrators of such violence. Special emphasis will be laid on programmes and measures to deal with trafficking in women and girls.

Support Services

The provision of support services for women, like childcare facilities, including creches at work places and educational institutions, homes for the aged and the disabled will be expanded and improved to create an enabling environment and to ensure their full cooperation in social, political and economic life. Women-friendly personnel policies will also be drawn up to encourage women to participate effectively in the developmental process.

Rights of the Girl Child

All forms of discrimination against the girl child and violation of her rights shall be eliminated by undertaking strong measures both preventive and punitive within and outside the family. These would relate specifically to strict enforcement of laws against prenatal sex selection and the practices of female foeticide, female infanticide, child marriage, child abuse, child prostitution, etc. Removal of discrimination in the treatment of the girl child within the family and outside and projection of a positive image of the girl child will be actively fostered. There will be special emphasis on the needs of the girl child and earmarking of substantial investments in areas relating to food and nutrition, health and education, and in vocational education. In implementing programmes for eliminating child labour, there will be special focus on girl children.

Mass Media

Media will be used to portray images consistent with human dignity of girls and women. The Policy will specifically strive to remove demeaning, degrading and negative conventional stereotypical images of women and violence against women. Private sector partners and media networks will be involved at all levels to ensure equal access for women particularly in the area of information and communication technologies. The media would be encouraged to develop codes of conduct, professional guidelines and other self-regulatory mechanisms to remove gender stereotypes and promote balanced portrayals of women and men.

Operational Strategies

Action Plans

The Plans will specifically include the following:

(i) Measurable goals to be achieved by 2010.
(ii) Identification and commitment of resources.
(iii) Responsibilities for implementation of action points.
(iv) Structures and mechanisms to ensure efficient monitoring, revise and gender impact assessment of action points and policies.
(v) Introduction of a gender perspective in the budgeting process.

In order to support better planning and programme formulation and adequate allocation of resources, Gender Development Indices (GDI) will be developed by networking with specialized agencies. These could be analyzed and studied in depth. Gender auditing and development of evaluation mechanisms will also be undertaken alongside.

The Plans of Action thus prepared will clearly specify:

(i) the measurable goals to be achieved along with the time targets, preferably in consonance with the time-frames set by the other women-related national policies;
(ii) commitment of resources;
(iii) earmarking of the benefits under WCP;
(iv) fixing of responsibilities for implementation of the Action Points; and
(v) identification of structures and mechanisms to ensure effective review, monitoring, and impact assessment of all the related policies, Plans of Action and programmes in raising the status of women, adolescent girls and girl children at par with their counterparts.

Institutional Mechanisms

Institutional mechanisms, to promote the advancement of women, which exist at the Central and State levels, will be strengthened. These will be through interventions as may be appropriate and will relate to, among others, provision of adequate resources, training and advocacy skills to effectively influence macropolicies, legislation, programmes, etc. to achieve the empowerment of women. National and State Councils are to be formed to oversee the operationalisation of the Policy on a regular basis. The National Council will be headed by the Prime Minister and the State Councils by the Chief Ministers and be broad in composition, having representatives from the concerned departments/ministries, National and State Commissions for Women, Social Welfare Boards, representatives of non-government organizations, women's organizations, corporate sector, trade unions, financing institutions, academics, experts, social activists, etc. These bodies will review the progress made in implementing the Policy twice a year. The Operational strategy, as prescribed in the Policy, directs all the Central Ministries and State Departments to draw up Time-Bound Action Plans for translating the Policy into a set of concrete actions through a participatory process of consultations with all concerned, both in the governmental and non-governmental sectors. Accordingly, the first step in this direction was preparation of a National Plan of Action for implementation of the Policy by the Nodal Department of Women and Child development through identifying its partners; specifying Action Points in all the women-related development sectors; developing an in-built mechanism for effective co-ordination and monitoring of the implementation of the Policy; besides evaluating/ assessing the impact of the implementation of Policy in improving the status of women, based on a Gender Development Index.

National and State Resources Centres on women will be established with mandates for collection and dissemination of information, undertaking research work, conducting surveys, implementing training and awareness generation programmes, etc. These Centres will link up with women's study centres schools of social work, home science colleges and other research and academic institutions through suitable information networking systems. While institutions at the district level will be strengthened, at the grassroots women will be helped by Government through its programmes to organise and strengthen into Self-Help Groups (SHGs) at the *anganwadi*/village/town level. The women's groups will be helped to institutionalise themselves into registered societies and to federate at the panchayat/municipal level. These societies will bring about synergistic implementation of all the social and economic development programmes by drawing resources made available through government and non-government channels, including banks and financial institutions and by establishing a close interface with the panchayats/ municipalities.

Resource Management

Availability of adequate financial, human and market resources to implement the Policy will be managed by concerned departments, financial credit institutions and banks, private sector, civil society and other connected institutions. This process will include:

(*a*) Assessment of benefits flowing to women and resource allocation to the programmes relating to them through an exercise of gender budgeting. Appropriate changes in policies will be made to optimise benefits to women under these schemes.

(*b*) Adequate resource allocation to develop and promote the policy outlined earlier based on (*a*) above by concerned departments.

(*c*) Developing synergy between personnel of Health, Rural Development, Education and Women and Child Development Department at field level and other village level functionaries.

(*d*) Meeting credit needs by banks and financial credit institutions through suitable policy initiatives and development of new institutions in coordination with the Department of Women and Child Development.

Legislation

The existing legislative structure will be reviewed and additional legislative measures taken by identified departments to implement the Policy. This will also involve a review of all existing laws including personal, customary and tribal laws, subordinate legislation, related rules as well as executive and administrative regulations to eliminate all gender discriminatory references. Effective implementation of legislation would be promoted by involving civil society and community. Appropriate changes in legislation will be undertaken, if necessary.

In addition, strict enforcement of all relevant legal provisions and speedy redressal of grievances will be ensured, with a special focus on violence and gender-related atrocities. Measures will also be undertaken to prevent and punish sexual harassment at the place of work, protection for women workers in the organised/unorganised sector and strict enforcement of relevant laws such as Equal Remuneration Act and Minimum Wages Act. Crimes against women, their incidence, prevention, investigation, detection and prosecution will be regularly reviewed at all crime review fora and conferences at the central, state and district levels. Recognised local, voluntary organizations will be authorised to lodge complaints and facilitate registration, investigations and legal proceedings related to violence and atrocities against girls and women. Women's Cells in police stations, women police stations, family courts, mahila courts, strengthened and expanded to eliminate violence and atrocities against women. Widespread dissemination of information will be done on all aspects of legal rights, human rights and other entitlements of women, through specially designed legal literacy programmes and rights information programmes.

Gender Sensitisation

Training of personnel of executive, legislative and judicial wings of the State, with a special focus on policy and programme framers, implementation and development agencies, law enforcement machinery and the judiciary, as well as non-governmental organizations will be undertaken. Other measures will include:

(*a*) promoting societal awareness to gender issues and women's human rights, review of curriculum and educational materials to include gender education and human rights issues, removal of all references derogatory to the dignity of women, and

(*b*) use of different forms of mass media to communicate social messages relating to women's equality and empowerment.

Panchayati Raj Institutions (PRIs)

The PRIs will play a central role in the process of enhancing women's participation in public life. The PRIs and the local self governments will be actively involved in the implementation and execution of the National Policy for Women at the grassroots level.

Partnership with voluntary sector organizations

The involvement of voluntary organizations, associations,

federations, trade unions, non-governmental organizations, women's organizations, as well as institutions dealing with education, training and research will be ensured in the formulation, implementation, monitoring and review of all policies and programmes affecting women. Towards this end, they will be provided with appropriate support related to resources and capacity building and facilitated to participate actively in the process of the empowerment of women.

International Cooperation

The Policy will aim at implementation of international obligations/commitments in all sectors on empowerment of women such as the Convention on All Forms of Discrimination Against Women (CEDAW), Convention on the Rights of the Child (CRC), International Conference on Population and Development (ICPD+5) and other such instruments. International, regional and sub-regional cooperation towards the empowerment of women will continue to be encouraged through sharing of experiences, exchange of ideas and technology, networking with institutions and organizations and through bilateral and multi-lateral partnerships.

The following measurable/monitorable goals having a direct bearing on the empowerment of women and the girl child, have also been adopted in the Action Plans:

- Reduction of poverty ratio by 5 percentage points by 2007 and by 15 percentage points by 2012;
- Providing gainful (high-quality) employment to the addition to the labour force over the Tenth Plan period;
- All children in school by 2003; all children to complete 5 years of schooling by 2007;
- Reduction of gender gaps in literacy and age rates by at least 50 per cent by 2007;
- Reduction in the decadal rate of population growth between 2001 and 2011 to 16.2 per cent;
- Increase in literacy rate to 75 per cent within the Plan period;
- Reduction of IMR to 45 per 1000 live births by 2007 and to 28 by 2012;

- Reduction of MMR to 2 per 1000 live births by 2007 and to 1 by 2012; and
- All villages to have sustained access to potable drinking water by 2007.

Acknowledging the fact that women's equality in power sharing and active participation in decision making, both in administrative and political spheres, is a very strong instrument to achieve the goals of empowerment, necessary steps have been initiated to guarantee equal access and full participation to women in decision-making bodies, including the legislative, executive, judicial, corporate, statutory bodies and their advisory commissions/committees, boards, etc. Affirmative action such as reservations/quotas, including in the higher political, administrative and legislative bodies may also be considered, if necessary, on a time-bound basis. Introduction of women-friendly personnel policies is an additional feature.

The process of organising women into SHGs to provide them a permanent fora for articulating their needs and contributing their perspectives to development, has been made for tremendous progress as it has already brought into action more than a million SHGs all over the country. Experience has shown that these Groups have been very effective institutions at the grassroot level in facilitating access to women, be it for financial or material resources or services or for information.

As much of the success of empowering women depends upon the holistic impact of various sectoral achievements, efforts will be initiated/intensified during converge the existing services, resources, infrastructure and manpower available both in the women-specific and women-related sectors with an ultimate objective of optimising the benefits with greater cost effectiveness. To this effect, efforts will be made to converge the services of health care, nutrition supplementation, safe drinking water, adult/functional/legal literacy, gainful employment both wage and self-employment, sanitation, health and nutrition awareness, knowledge and information about management of diseases, counselling towards safe motherhood practices, nutrition, welfare services, etc. Governmental institutions and efforts by themselves alone are not adequate in terms of human and financial resources to achieve empowerment/advancement of women in its various dimensions. Therefore, they need to be supplemented by Civil Society organizations (voluntary organizations). Already, a large number of such organizations have emerged throughout the country, and some of them have made significant contribution towards projecting and addressing women's issues at the grassroot levels. Also, as corporate bodies have a strategic interface with the working people, their services are to be utilized for gender sensitisation of the corporate world as a whole, including their work force. Efforts are also on to draw upon their infrastructure and resources for the implementation of women's development programmes, besides ensuring that their employment practices adhere to the norms of social and gender justice.

Finally, the Tenth Plan will also take cognisance of the gender asymmetry in the population pyramid with 'males outnumbering females' as a whole and 'females outnumbering males' at the upper end of the age structure and calls for urgent interventions to protect the girl child, besides providing social security for the aged women. The special interventions launched through the *Balika Samriddhi Yojana* (BSY) in 1999 do not seem to make the desired impact on the conditions of the adolescent/girl child who is still a victim of various types of discrimination, both within and outside the family. It is hoped that the National Population Policy, with its much-advocated strategy of concentrating on the 133 high fertility districts identified specially for the purpose of paying special attention on population of time.

While the above-mentioned holistic strategies are expected to reinforce the ongoing process of empowering women, the Tenth Plan also suggests a sector-specific three-fold strategy for empowering women through; (i) Social Empowerment, (ii) Economic Empowerment, and (iii) Gender Justice, as per the following details.

COMMITMENTS OF THE TENTH PLAN TO EMPOWER WOMEN

The Approach

To continue with the major strategy of empowering women as agents of social change and development.

Strategies

To adopt a sector-specific **3-fold strategy for empowering women**, based on the prescriptions of the National Policy for Empowerment of Women. This strategy includes:

Social Empowerment—to create an enabling environment through various affirmative developmental policies and programmes for development of women, besides providing them easy and equal access to all the basic minimum services so as to enable them to realize their full potentials.

Economic Empowerment—to ensure provision of training, employment and income-generation activities with both 'forward' and 'backward' linkages with the ultimate objective of making all potential women economically independent and self-reliant.

• **Gender Justice**—to eliminate all forms of gender discrimination and thus, allow women to enjoy not only the *de jure* but also the *de facto* rights and fundamental freedom at par with men in all spheres, viz. political, economic, social, civil, cultural, etc.

COMMENTS AND GAPS IN NPEW

The goal of National Policy for the Empowerment of Women (2001) is to bring about the advancement, development and empowerment of women. The policy gives prescriptions for positive socio-economic policies, equal access to participate in decision making, equal access to health, education, employment, strengthening the legal system, mainstreaming gender perspective in the development, etc. In spite of Constitutional provisions, legal safeguards as also ratification of various United Nations conventions, policies, Platform For Action, plan programmes, policies and planned programmes, the desired results for gender equality have not been achieved.

So, there is a widespread gap between government intentions and actions in all sectors of development. Even some of the states have yet to prepare and finalise a state-specific policy and action plan based on the NPEW enunciated by Government of India and action plan thereof.

Institutional mechanisms for the advancement of women suffer from inadequate financial and human resources confronting national machineries, lack of understanding of gender equality and of gender mainstreaming, prevailing gender stereotypes and discriminatory attitudes as also competing government priorities and insufficient links to civil society. Many schemes in the Department of Women and Child Development, Government of India (GOI) and other ministries have been initiated. Effective evaluation has not been done about their impact on women's lives. The only achievement is change in the names of some of the schemes of GOI such as *Indira Mahila Yojana,* Integrated Women's Empowerment Project, *Swayam Sidha, Swa-shakti,* etc. The *Balika Samridhi Yojana* is also on the verge of dismantling. The State Women Development Corporations in many states face a resource crunch and many of their units have been closed down. In spite of Government commitment on various platforms, the Department of Women and Child Development has not been able to set up a National Resource Centre for Women, which has been reflected in its various annual reports.

NGOs' support and benefits through public programmes have given voice to grassroots women that the gap between acceptance of women's needs and recommendations and actual policy and programmes remains virtually unbridgeable. However, the women's movement has been a powerful instrument in bringing about improvements in the right of women; in enforcing rights already granted to them; and in highlighting serious gaps in many legal provisions and procedures; for monitoring of the actual status of women in several sectors through research and data on women for employment, income, health, education, legal help has recorded that progress is patchy at best and dismal at worst, going by the Human Development Report on gender indices for our country. Further, the provision of credit, offering of special subsides and schemes for deprived groups seems to have made little difference in the absence of institutional changes which in turn cannot be implemented unless they are grounded in the local, social and political matrix. It is not enough to ensure credit adequacy alone, but also access to it and its benefits have to spread widely enough to contribute to increasing the overall productivity for the well-being of the people engaged in it.

Though women form a critical component of the labour force in agriculture, the latest Census data lends evidence of a sharp rise in the female work participation rates in the rural areas from 22.3 per cent in 1991 to 25.7 per cent in 2001. Even this does not reflect the real extent of women's labour. Substantial numbers of womenheaded households are also not even recognized so far. This also points towards the conclusion that none of the programmes—whether it is credit access or extension schemes for technology dissemination—have especially benefited women. A large number of indicators shows that the structural, institutional and organisational changes under way push women farther to the fringes of the formal economy. This is also clear from the studies of green revolution economies which reflected that the introduction of technology which makes work easier in traditional occupations considered the woman's domain inevitably pushes women out of those jobs. There is also growing evidence from a number of countries that the opening up of international trade in commodities and farm products leads to marginalized women in the formal production system. Women are now moving from wage worker to casual worker, depending on domestic and family compulsions. The shift towards agricultural exports and away from food crops to cash crops is a serious threat to food security of women.

There has been no feminization of labour as argued by some. Much of the female labour has entered into traditional female occupations which have become increasingly casual/ temporary/insecure with poor rewards. Even the organized sector has resorted to such strategies to turn skilled female labour into casual labour. The new economic developments are not promoting labour-intensive technologies or capital-intensive technologies. Large industries opt for capital-intensive production to become 'competitive'. This assumption that it is necessary to invest in human capital—education and health—is also not valid. Physical capital and productive assets are not generated by inappropriate policies, and redistribution, the well-being of the majority is unlikely to be taken care of. For example, data indicates that small landholdings have higher income per hectare and have an incentive to reduce birth rate. In this context, gender skewness, 'women's development' will take a back seat. Further, benefits of the growing global economy have been unevenly distributed, creating wider economic disparities, unsafe work environments and perpetuating gender inequality in the informal economy and rural sector. Women with comparable skills to men lag behind men in income and career mobility in the formal sector.

Income inequality, unemployment and levels of poverty of the most vulnerable groups (rural and poor women), contribute to the widening economic gap between men and women. The structural adjustment policies and the process of globalisation, in particular, have been especially painful to specific groups such as the poor and marginalized women, peasant women and women workers of the unorganized sector. Social sector expenditure and public investment have been slashed. Real per capita spending on the social sector infrastructure covering housing, health and sanitation has fallen sharply. In urban centres, declining male employment has led to an increase in casual employment. This makes for insecurity and reduced incomes. There have been schemes for aiding women in microenterprises but these are ad hoc programmes. Some women narrate harrowing stories of how they have to run from pillar to post for micro-credit, which has been hailed as a great achievement. No doubt they represent women's thrift potential and self-help groups do assist poor women.

There has been a plethora of schemes for rural employment but little impact on women's lives. Women as producers in farm and forestry are not represented in forest personnel.

Women do not also get sufficient information on what they can collect, and get hauled up by forest officials. Fuel substitutes like *gobar* (bio) gas or solar cookers have not become real alternatives because of their high cost and poor maintenance. Smokeless *chulhas* (stoves) have run into rough weather because of bad planning and design inappropriate to women's cooking practices.

Not only this, even institutional change being brought about for limited purposes often influences other changes, e.g., self-help groups are operational as micro-credit enterprises often with linkages to institutions such as NABARD to expand credit flows to the sector have been found to promote political mobilization among women. Gender perspective, extension service schemes for 'diversification and modernisation of agricultural practices' have not evidently been linked to credit operations. Further, environmental policies and programmes lack a gender perspective. These are inadequate to account for women's roles and contributions to environmental sustainability. The low presence of few women in the formulation and implementation of environmental policy and their under-representation in decision-making bodies are aggravating factors.

The government cites the National Crime Records Bureau figures to accept that crimes against women have increased, but says it has taken several measures to deal with the problem—like setting up all-women police stations in 14 states and strengthening present laws, an exercise undertaken by the National Commission for Women (NCW). The government paper does not mention that most states now want to close down these "ineffective" police stations while the NCW's 200-odd recommendations, including amendments to laws on dowry and trafficking, have virtually been ignored. There is lack of proper understanding of the root causes of violence against women and inadequacy of data on the various forms of violence hinders efforts. Socio-cultural attitudes and values reinforce women's subordinate place in society. Improving the response of legal officials, especially criminal justice officials, is weak in many states, while prevention strategies remain fragmented and reactive, sustained efforts are missing for advocacy against violence as also bills pending before the Standing Committee of Parliament. The philosophy on the basis of which Family Courts have been established is to treat problems relating to family (divorce, maintenance, alimony, custody, education and family support to children) as a social therapeutic problem rather than legal. Family Courts are yet to be set up in all states as also in all districts. Integration of Support Services with Family Courts are far from satisfactory to enable these courts to actualise their goal and bring about attitudinal changes in the spouses to achieve speedy justice to make a family happy and not to disrupt family life.

Discriminatory legislations exist, and family, civil and penal codes are still not fully gender sensitive. Women have little exposure to law, legal literacy and resources. In view of insensitivity and gender discrimination of the law enforcement machinery and the judiciary, and the perpetuation of traditional and stereotypical attitudes, there has been frequent violation of women's human rights which continues unabated in some of the states. Laws require review and amendment and need to be framed with a view to securing, promoting and enforcing women's human rights at all levels of public and private spheres. The enactment of legislation on prevention of domestic violence to women to address the wide spread problem of domestic violence against women and to create an institution of protection officers for protection of women from domestic violence is still pending for approval. Similarly, the Bill on Sexual Harassment of Women at the Workplace is not introduced as promised. Thus, mounting violence against women is another alarming signal that the elimination of the subordinate status of women is not as easily overcome as we think, and underestimate the strength of patriarchy and caste politics.

The rhetoric of empowerment is enabling women to become victims of oppressors who should be brought to book. Our judges and lawyers, the police and the criminal justice system in most of the cases fail to give justice to women victims, and the offenders are acquitted most of the time. Policy and its implementation have made many prescriptions is different directions. Many new responsibilities have been added without any reduction in the basic set of deprivations or work burdens; employment and education are becoming tools for family welfare. Ideally, these should have been women's source of freedom: birth control is manipulation for population control rather than relieving women from reproductive burdens.

Domestic responsibilities often prevent the girl child from pursuing her education. Programmes are hindered by a lack of financial and human resources, statistical data disaggregated by sex and technical capacity. There was little established national machinery to implement policies and programmes for the girl child. The girls' and women's education was accepted as important all along and there were recommendations related to training of more women teachers, curriculum, etc. but there was no appreciation of the fact that the supply of books, uniforms and free education in schools and teachers was not enough to induce parents to send girls to school and retain them there. The missing steps are: inadequate hostels for girls and those that do exist are of a poor standard; very little is done to gear up the positive interventionist role of education so that the educational curriculum is even today dominated by academic thrusts and market-led courses. Traditionally assigned gender roles circumscribe women's choices in education and careers and compel women to assume the burden for household responsibilities. Initiatives and programmes aimed at women's increased participation in decision making are hindered by a lack of human and financial resources for training and advocacy for political careers, and accountability of elected officials for promoting gender equality and women's participation in public life. Despite vigorous campaigning by women's groups, and despite the state's commitment to increasing women's political participation, all political parties have been more than reluctant to field women candidates. The Women's Reservation Bill which promises one-third representation to women in parliament, has yet to be tabled for discussion while parties have made a commitment on paper.

Women's Studies Centres and cells may be doing good work, but they lack proper leadership and adequate resources. Poor infrastructure and insufficient resources have made their tasks difficult and ineffective. State governments are to provide support once the University Grants Commission (UGC) grants run out. In general, there is a lack of broader perspective and imagination, insufficient autonomy and stranglehold of university bureaucracy, tardy and erratic release of funds by the UGC and, to cap it all, a low status for Women's Studies within the academia. A major gap is still found in the narrow discipline concentration among women in higher education. Concern has been expressed in many committees and by women's groups on the importance of increasing the presence of women in science and technology and in professional streams. Considering that the bulk of technological advances have never addressed women's work and the enormous drudgery it involves, one is wrong in asking that in the present some of it may be eased.

Thus, it is a misnomer to call the Department of Women and Child Development, Government of India's National Policy for the Empowerment of Women a 'policy'. The document is disappointing because it betrays no knowledge of all that has happened on the women's front in the aftermath of the economic reforms and is a series of ad hoc suggestions made many times before. It is an overload of laudable 'intentions' but lacks any kind of vision. The onus is put on women to empower themselves and there is very little by way of policy goals or implementing strategies that will create conditions for gender equality. It has nothing to say on the International Labour Organization (ILO) convention on home workers not being ratified by India. 'Women are expected to participate in decision-making. However, while the issues on which they would like to decide move outside the jurisdiction of these decisions, the right-wing politics has made it harder for women to act on a united front. In respect of health policy, the same battle has been going on to gear the healthcare system to promote women's well-being and not be obsessed solely with their 'mother' role. If this interest in the mother had really received adequate attention, we would not have one of the highest figures of maternal mortality and a poor gender development index. Absence of a holistic approach to health care for women and girls throughout the life cycle has further exacerbated by absence of gender-sensitive health research and technology, data disaggregated by sex and age, and user-friendly indicators. A shortage of financial and human resources has led to inadequate infrastructure and service delivery.

REFERENCES

Government of India. (2001). Planning Commission. (2002). Tenth Five-Year Plan, New Delhi.

Government of India, Ministry of Agriculture. (1979–80). Report of the National Committee on Role and Participation of Women in Agriculture and Rural Development, New Delhi.

Government of India, Ministry of Education and Social Welfare, Department of Social Welfare. (1974). Towards Equality—Report of the Committee on the Status of Women in India, New Delhi.

Government of India, Ministry of Human Resource Development. (2001). National Policy for the Empowerment of Women, New Delhi.

Government of India, Ministry of Human Resource Development, Department of Women and Child Development. (1988). National Perspective Plan for Women. (1988–2000 A.D), New Delhi.

Government of India, Ministry of Human Resource Development, Department of Women and Child Development. (1995). Country Report, Fourth World Conference in Beijing, New Delhi.

Government of India, Ministry of Human Resource Development, Department of Women and Child Development. (2002–03). Annual Report.

Government of India, Ministry of Human Resource Development, Department of Women and Child Development. (1987). Report of National Expert Committee on Women Prisoners, New Delhi.

Government of India, Ministry of Human Resource Development, Department of Women's Welfare. (1985). Nairobi Forward Looking Strategies for the Advancement of Women, New Delhi.

Government of India, Ministry of Human Resource Development, Department of Women and Child Development. (1988). Empowered Girl, Empowered Society, New Delhi.

Government of India, Ministry of Human Resource Development, Department of Women and Child Development. (1999). Schemes for Assistance—A Handbook, New Delhi.

Government of India, Ministry of Human Resource Development, Department of Women and Child Development. (1993). Policies and Programmes for the Advancement of Women, New Delhi.

Government of India, Ministry of Human Resource Development, Department of Women and Child Development. (1988). *Shram Shakti*—Report of National Commission of Self Employed Women, New Delhi.

Katyal, A. (2000). Government NGOs differ over women's status : *The Times of India News Service, Times of India.*

National Commission for Women. (1990–2001). A Decade of Endeavour, Volume II.

Sen, M.K. and Shiva Kumar, A.K. (2001). Women in India—How Free? How Equal?: United Nations.

United Nations. (2000). Action for Gender Equality and the Advancement of Women.

United Nations. (2000). Convention on the Elimination of all Forms of Discrimination against Women.

United Nations, Department of Public Information. (2001). Platform for Action and the Beijing Declaration: Fourth World Conference on Women. (1995). New York.

Chapter 2

Women, Work and Empowerment

Kamla Sankaran

The participation of women in the work force has been on the increase internationally in the recent past. These changes have raised important issues for policy makers in several countries including India, who deal with increasing number of women in the labour force, most of whom are in the unorganized sector of the economy.

However, in the case of India, the results of the labour force surveys published by International Labour Organization (ILO) and the census of India do not point to any marked increase in the labour force participation rates of women; and in fact showed a decline in the 1990s as compared to the 1970s and 1980s. While the female labour force participation rate was 16.9 in the census of 1971, it rose to 27.1 in 1981 and fell to 23.4 in 1991. The National Sample Survey (NSS) 55th round survey for 1993–94 revealed "a near stagnation in the number of women workers in the country as a whole and near absolute reduction in the number of women workers in rural India". This reduction in the number of women workers in rural India, by a little over 1.3 million, is just about offset by a rise in the number of urban women workers (1.4 million).

According to the 1991 Census, the total workforce in India was estimated to be 317 million. Of this, 91.5 per cent of the labour force was employed in the unorganized sector. The percentage of women in the unorganized sector is proportionally greater than men as 95.8 per cent of women in the labour force are in the unorganized sector. Recent NSS data shows that the work force was around 397 million persons in India in 1999–2000, of which 123 million are women workers. Also recent NSSO data indicate that the trend of slower growth in the organized sector employment vis-à-vis unorganized sector employment continued in the 1990s. A larger number of respondents reported themselves as casual employees, their numbers rose to 33 per cent in 1999–2000 as compared with 30 per cent in 1987–88. There has also been a corresponding decline in the number of those who reported themselves as self-employed while the number of those who are salaried remained more or less constant in this regard. Corresponding to these trends, we also note that there is very slow growth in employment in organized sector. This is reflected in the small growth in the number of employees i.e., 0.48 per cent between 1980 and 1998.

Women and Work

There are many activities that can be classified as 'work'. There has been intense debate in India about what constitutes work and what merits being included in the national statistics as being productive or economically meaningful. This debate has to be understood in the broader backdrop of patriarchal prejudices which define what kinds of activity are 'work' and hence can be included as being productive or economically important. Women's work performed in the home often gets relegated as unimportant, or being for self consumption by family members or failing in the category of care giving and therefore not 'work'.

Until the 1981 Census, 'work' was defined as 'participation in any economically productive activity'. This therefore excluded activities performed particularly by women, for consumption within the family. The 1991 Census defined work as participation in any economically productive activity, whether the participation is physical or mental. An added feature of this census was that activities like cultivation for self-consumption and unpaid work for family enterprises were also considered to be work. The National Sample Survey enumerates all activities pursued for pay, profit or family gain. In the agricultural sector activities geared to the market as well as non-market are included. Yet even this definition is not capable of capturing the unpaid domestic work performed by women that may not amount to 'work' as defined above. In fact, the Time Utilization Survey reveal that women spend nearly ten times the amount of time spent by men towards their unpaid family responsibilities.

Although the definition of work has been refined and the extent of women's work which is not enumerated is less than in the past, capturing the data accurately is not easy. The assumption that the nature of economic activity for men as well as women is similar leads to problems. Women, more often than men, combine economic and domestic work. Differentiating the economic work of women from their domestic work poses problems. Besides the inadequate definition, the inaccuracies of data collection also leads to under enumeration. Often respondents speak on behalf of the women and may give inaccurate responses regarding the work done by women. The biases and perceptions of the surveys may also lead to inaccuracies in the information. Adding to the problems of inadequate definition are the difficulties in assigning accurate economic value to the non market-related work of women.

Women are more likely to be either self employed or casual workers as compared to men. While 42% of the urban male workers in 1993 were in regular salaried employment, the figure was only 28% in the case of women. The greater share of women workers in casual and contract employment is also borne out through case studies. Thus women's position in the labour market is more adverse than that of men.

There is a great variety of the nature of work performed by women in the unorganized (or informal) sector in India. The common feature of the work performed by women is that they are low paid and under valued. It has been noted that women's earnings as compared to men's reflect an earnings gap in India. This is despite the fact that occupational segregation by sex is lower in countries in Asia as compared to the rest of the world. The gender gap in earnings and the persistent payment for lower wages in jobs where women are employed has been a source of concern. The nature of work is also changing. There is an increase in the demand for flexible, part-time subcontract work indicating the semi informalization of the formal sector. Many of these newer jobs have been in the form of home-based work particularly involving women workers. International conferences and reports are increasingly focusing attention on the need to combat various forms of discrimination in the fields of employment. The platform of action adopted by the 1995 Beijing Conference of Women called for "elimination of occupational segregation and all forms of employment segregation" (Strategic objective F5) and to "guarantee the rights of women and men to equal pay for work of equal value" (para 165 of platform).

There is a great diversity in the nature of work and employment relations for the millions of persons in the unorganized sector (which includes home-based workers) in India. The recent standards relating to home work and part-time work adopted by the ILO and attempts to formulate standards on contract work, in the latter half of the 1990s, is an acknowledgement that the nature of work is changing internationally.

What is the unorganized sector?

NSSO data reveal that the majority Indian labour force works in what has come to be known (in India) as the unorganized sector. The unorganized sector is an important contributor to the Net Domestic product (NDP) contributing over 60 per cent to the NDP.

The unorganized sector includes agricultural labour, rural workers engaged in animal husbandry and livestock rearing, workers engaged in cottage and village industries, rural artisans, weavers, fishermen, leather workers and those working in tanneries, workers engaged in collecting forest produce, collecting tendu leaves, workers in brick kilns, workers engaged in stone quarries, building and construction workers, *beedi* workers, workers engaged in the timber and felling industries mills, salt workers among other categories and petty traders/vendors domestic workers and those engaged in home-based work.

Commentators have noted that the unorganized sector would include all those in the labour force who are not in the organized sector. The organized sector usually covers establishment in the public sector and those in the private sector employing ten or more workers. This also corresponds with those establishments covered by legislation.

The unorganized sector is characterized by low wages and where conditions of work are often outside the sphere of legislative protection. Work conditions are precarious and uncertain and made more so by the reasons that they may fall outside legislative protection at the present time. This is because in the Indian context the 'protection' afforded by the labour law is not uniformly available to all those in wage employment. Labour law excluded a large number of workers (notwithstanding attempts by courts to liberally construe labour statutes) with the coverage of the laws restricted to certain large establishments in the organized/formal sector employing a minimum number of employees. The legal framework for regulating employment relationships is largely focused on "typical" full-time regular employment in the formal sector. In addition, the workers in the unorganized sector are also non-unionized. This further contributes to their vulnerability and relative lack of 'voice' and therefore their invisibility.

CURRENT CHALLENGES

Globalization has posed new challenges to women working in both the organized and unorganized sector. There is a documented threat of "loss of employment without creation of any new employment". Loss of city space where street vendors could carry out their activities, loss of livelihood reported by those producing yarn due to the introduction of imported yarn or silk, loss of fishing catch due to deep-sea trawlers, flooding into the country of cheaper imports due to liberalization have all led to loss of traditional employments and livelihood. While policies need to be framed to increase employment and livelihood opportunities for women, efforts must also be made that such jobs are capable of providing 'decent work' for the women concerned.

The coverage of labour laws at the present time typically excludes workers in the unorganized sector. This needs to be remedied. The Unorganized Workers Bill currently being discussed in the country requires political consensus to be enacted into law. Until recently, even trade unions in the organized sector had marginalized concerns of the unorganized sector workers. This is slowly but surely changing.

In the organized sector, the effect of casualization has been to push more women into the unorganized sector with its typically low-paid jobs. The Exports Processing Zones and Exports Oriented Units that have newly been set up have been a major employer of women workers. Yet the denial, or at least the systematic non-observance of labour laws in these areas has been a cause of concern. There is thus a pressing need to revamp the labour laws enforcement system in the country. The low levels of inspections and the fairly blatant violation of labour laws has been a matter of concern. Extension and enforcement of protective labour laws that benefit women need to be addressed if the working conditions of women workers need to be ameliorated. Special focus needs to be given to inspection of premises in the unorganized sector. Adequate number of labour law enforcement personnel should be women and they should be sensitized to the working conditions of women workers.

In order to improve their working conditions and status, women workers should be encouraged to join organizations that present and defend their interests. These organizations could take a variety of forms: trade unions, *mahila mandals*, self-help groups and cooperatives. Many of these organizations not only serve as organizations representing interests of women workers, they can also have the ability of advancing the employment and business interests of women workers particularly in the case of women who engage in small levels of self-employed activity—arranging for micro credit, social security services, insurance, etc. The Self Employed Women's Association (SEWA) could serve as a prime example of what such a multi-faceted trade union could achieve for its numbers.

Skills development for workers, particularly women who work in the unorganized sector, has been a concern for policy makers. Agriculture that employs the largest number of persons, is a much-neglected area. Extension services in the areas of livestock, soil conservation, and other related occupations can augment the livelihood of women in these sectors.

There has been a demand and pressure for liberalizing the present laws that prohibit night work for women in those sectors that are fast opening up. These would include sectors such as electronics, information technology, food processing, agro industry and textiles. These are sectors that either require continuous processing to prevent deterioration of raw materials (as in the case of food processing) or may include back office outsourcing establishment that takes advantage of the information and communication technology to provide greater employment to both men and women. These have been areas where demands for night work for women on the grounds of prevention of discrimination have been raised. In India, women who work in factories and offices are prohibited from working at night. The Factories Act adopted in 1948 stated that no woman should be required or allowed to work in any factory except between the hours of 6.00 a.m. and 7.00 p.m. with the proviso that the hours may be varied provided that no woman may work between 10.00 p.m. to 5.00 a.m. However, the law itself provides ways in which this ban on night work for women can be circumvented. The Section states that the State Government may make rules providing for the exemption from the ban on night work of women in fish curing or fish canning factories, where the employment of women during night hours is necessary to prevent damage to, or deterioration of any raw material. This exemption can be subject to such conditions as the Government deems necessary.

The National Commission on Labour, appointed by the

Government of India to look into several labour questions, has recommended that the ban on night work by women can be lifted if the number of women workers per shift in an establishment is not less than five, and if the management is able to provide satisfactory arrangements for their transport, safety and rest after or before shift hours. The matter is currently pending a final legislative decision. If permitted, it is expected that night work would open further avenues of employment for women. Yet, there is also an urgent need to take into account the high degrees of violence that women face on the street while travelling to work, poor public transport facilities and the levels of sexual harassment at the workplace that can be expected to increase if night work is permitted.

The lack of adequate social security for women workers has been increasingly voiced. Article 38 of the Constitution of India mandates the State to promote the welfare of the people by securing and protecting a social order in which justice—social, economic and political—shall guide all institutions. Articles 41 states that the State shall, within the limits of its economic capacity, add to public assistance in the case of unemployment, old age, sickness and disabled, and other cases of undeserved want. Article 42 requires that the State should make provisions for securing just and humane conditions of work and maternity relief while Article 47 mandates that the state shall raise the level of nutrition and the standard of living and provides basic social security to all citizens of India. Yet laws that provide social security to workers continue to barely apply to workers in the organized sector. As correctly summarized by the National Commission on Labour, "The problem is more acute for women workers. They lay (down) a triple role of a worker, housewife and mother. The lack of capital and assets, low and irregular income aided by frequent accidents, sickness and other contingencies, poor working and living conditions, low bargaining power and lack of outside linkages and opportunities for skills upgradation—all these interlinked factors drag women into deprivation, trapping them in the vicious circle of poverty. There is thus an urgent to set up welfare boards for working in different sectors. The state of Kerala already has in place such diverse boards that have the capacity to deliver social security benefits to lakhs of workers in the unorganized sector. This example could well be replicated across the country. Provident funds schemes that have been successfully extended to lakhs of workers in the *beedi* sector could also be another example of such extension of social security and welfare benefits.

In recent years, several issues have been raised questioning the need for protective legislation for women. While these have been raised in the context of the debate to remove restriction on night work for women, it cannot be denied that, given women's weaker economic and social position, reliance on law continues to be critical. A theme being increasingly highlighted is the need to review such protective legislation while keeping in mind that effective laws protecting women must honour the fine line ensuring safe working conditions for all workers, including women in the informal sector and providing equal opportunities for all workers seeking employment.

REFERENCES

Economic Growth, Employment Generation and Fundamental Principles and Rights at Work, co-authored with TCA Anant. (2003). Background Paper presented at ILO-CIE Conference on Globalization, Decent work and the ILO Declaration on Fundamental Principles and Right at Work, Kolkata, February.

Standing, G. (1998). 'Global Feminization Through Flexible Labour : A Theme Revisited', *World Development*, 27 (3).

Jeemol, U. (2001). Gender and Informality in Labour Market in South Asia. *Economic and Political Weekly*, Vol. 26 (26) 2360.

Sundaram, K. (2001). *Economic and Political Weekly*, Vol. 36, (34) August.

Vanamala, M. (2001). Information and Feminizaion of a Formal Sector Industry. A Case Study, *Economic and Political Weekly*, June.

Report on the Study Group on Women and Child Labour. (2002). National Commission on Labour, pp. 27–28, 33, 37, 80.

See Factories Act 1948 and the Shops and Establishment Act of different states. Women working in hospitals and in agriculture are exempt from such laws. This has been struck down as unconstitutional in a recent case by the Madras High Court *Vasantha R. v. Union of India* 2001 II LLJ 843 (Mad). The case was decided by the Madras High Court.

See Factories Act 1948, s 66(2). For instance the rules made under this Act in the state of Tamil Nadu provide that no woman shall be employed before 6 a.m. or after 7 p.m. for more than three days in a week; and no woman shall be employed after 11 p.m. and before 5 a.m. The number of days on which a woman may be so employed cannot exceed fifty days in a year.

See National Policy for the Empowerment of Women 2001 and Report of the Study Group on Women and Child Labour, National Commission on Labour. (2002).

See report of the National Commission on Labour 2002 available at http://www.labour.nic.in. Unlike countries in Europe who have denounced certain International Labour Conventions (C41 and C89) on the basis that women do not require protection except in cases of pregnancy and maternity; trade unions in India argue that there is a need to continue to prohibit night work of women. Since factories employing women are in the export sector, it is argued that the demand for permitting night work is driven by the need to have a third shift rather than an assessment of women worker's real position in the workplace.

The Equal Remuneration Act, 1976 in India mandates that men and women should be paid equal wages for 'same or similar work'. The ILO's Equal Remuneration Convention 1951 (No. 100) uses the concept of equal pay for work of equal value.

Chapter 3

Women's Empowerment Through Micro-credit

Zubair Meenai

A great deal of evidence from around the world indicates that gender inequalities undermine the effectiveness of development policies. It is seen that despite progress, gender disparities persist around the world. For example,

- In no region do women and men have equal rights. In a number of countries, women still lack independent access to land, manage property, conduct business, or even travel without their husband's consent;
- Women continue to have a systematically poorer command over a range of productive resources, including land, information and financial resources;
- Despite considerable increase in women's education relative to men, women continue to have limited opportunities and earn less than men in the labour market even when they have the same education and work experience as men;
- Women remain vastly underrepresented in politics and policy-making. They hold less than 10 per cent of the seats in parliament in most regions and less than 8 per cent in government ministerial positions (King & Mason, 2001).

As pointed out by a recent report (Sen & Kumar, 2001) commissioned by the office of the United Nations Resident

Coordinator in India, women in India:

- Are outnumbered by men—estimated 39 million missing women
- Face nutritional discrimination
- Have little control over own fertility and reproductive health
- Are less literate with higher dropout rates
- Work longer hours than men; their work is largely undervalued and unrecognized
- Earn lower wages for same work
- Are underrepresented in governance and decision making
- Are legally discriminated against in land and property rights
- Face violence inside and outside family throughout their lives.

WOMEN AND WORK

Women have extensive workloads with dual responsibility for farm and household production. Their work is getting harder and more time-consuming due to ecological degradation and changing agricultural technologies and practices. Women also have an active role and extensive involvement in livestock production, forest resource use and fishery processing and contribute considerably to household income through farm and non-farm activities as well as through work as landless agricultural labourers. However, women's work as family labour is underestimated and there are high degrees of inter-state and intra-state variations in gender roles in agriculture, environment and rural production.

As per the 1991 Census, the Indian work force participation rate is 37.7 per cent out of which the rate for women is 22.7 per cent, which is less than half the rate of 51.6 per cent for men. "The pattern of women's participation in the labour force varies across the country depending upon geographic region, caste, socio-economic class and formal and informal sectors. The rural female participation rate is 27.2 per cent, nearly thrice as much as the urban female participation rate of 9.7 per cent.

The percentage of labourers employed as main workers is higher among men than among women. In the case of marginal workers, this proportion is larger among women than among men. The majority of the main workers (66.8%) are employed in agricultural and allied industrial sectors. The proportion of women employed in this sector is 80.7 per cent, compared to 62.7 per cent for men. In rural areas, 89.5 per cent of the total females employed are engaged in the agricultural and allied industrial sector. In urban areas manufacturing, processing, servicing and repair, when it is in the household, absorb larger proportions of the total female employment compared to men. The reverse is true when it is other than household work. Industries which employ more women than men are *bidi* and match manufacturing, cotton textiles, cotton spinning, cashewnut processing, tobacco stemming and re-drying, canning, preserving and fish processing" (www.fao.org).

As is evident, rural Indian women are extensively involved in agricultural activities, their roles ranging from managers to landless labourers. In farm production, women's average contribution is estimated at 55 per cent to 66 per cent of the total labour with percentages much higher in certain regions (Venkateswaran, 1992). Livestock plays a major role in the rural households' economy. It provides draught power for the farm, manure for crops, energy for cooking and food for household consumption as well as the market. Women have a multiple role in this activity. It is known that women take care of animal production, their activities ranging from care of animals, grazing, fodder collection, cleaning of animal sheds to processing milk and livestock products. Similarly, indoor jobs like milking, feeding, cleaning, etc. are done by women. In the Indian Himalayas a pair of bullocks works 1064 hours, a man 1212 hours and a woman 3485 hours in a year on a one-hectare farm, a figure that illustrates women's significant contribution to agricultural production (www.fao.org).

Women also provide bulk of the labour in rice cultivation, and in the plantation sector also, women are the crucial labourers. Depending on the region and crops, women's contributions vary but they provide labour from planting to harvesting and post-harvest operations. In general, it is understood that women in tribal households enjoy more decision-making power than women in many other Indian households because of their greater contribution to household income.

Women accounted for 93 per cent of total employment in dairy production (World Bank, 1991). Depending upon the economic status, women perform the tasks of collecting fodder and collecting and processing dung. Women undertake dung composting and carrying it to the fields. Women also prepare cooking fuel by mixing dung with twigs and crop residues. Though women play a significant role in livestock management and production, women's control over livestock and its products is negligible. Rural Indian women are also intensively involved with the forests, their roles ranging from gathering, wage employment, production in farm forestry, etc. Women are the major gatherers and users of a much more diverse range of forest products than men.

Credit and Poverty: Since the late 1970s there has been increasing realization, that one of the obstacles preventing the poor from improving their lives was the lack of access to financial services. Attempts have therefore been made to develop more sustainable and reachable financial systems, than the previous schemes of direct credit. To meet women's expressed need for improved access to credit, particularly to small loans which allow them to engage in risk-averse, multi-production strategies and thereby to improve the livelihoods of their families, thrift and credit or 'self-help groups' (SHGs) have been promoted, both by the government as well as NGOs and donors. These groups initially draw on their own accumulated savings to provide loans to their members, and later link with the formal credit system to access funds, overcoming the limitations of their own resources.

Micro finance: Micro-finance arose in the 1980s as a response to doubts and research findings about state delivery of subsidized credit to poor farmers. In the 1970s, government agencies were the predominant channels of providing productive credit to those with no previous access to credit facilities, those who had been forced to pay usurious interest rates or were subject to rent seeking behaviour (Ledgerwood, 1998). Since the 1980s, the field of micro-finance has grown substantially. *The Grameen Bank* in Bangladesh developed highly effective techniques like taking services to the village level, promoting and motivating groups of the poor, use of group guarantees, compulsory savings mobilization, intensive supervision of borrowers, and decentralized and cost-effective operations, for lending to the poor (McGuire and Conroy, 2000).

The Micro-Credit Summit in Washington DC in February 1997, attended by some 1500 organizations from 137 countries, including a number of heads of states, helped focus attention on micro-credit. The declaration of the Summit stated that:

> *"There now exists both a substantial track record of accomplishments and a significant body of scholarly studies that together paint a picture of micro-credit as a compelling anti-poverty and development strategy. Taken together, these accomplishments communicate the possibility of moving toward a world freed from the blight of poverty within a length of time measured in years rather than decades or centuries* (MicroCredit Summit, 1997)."

Some major findings from practical experiences and other evaluative studies also pointed out the potential of micro-credit to help the poorest:

- Very poor people are a good credit risk, especially in the context of mutual responsibility systems
- Sustainability of programmes in the developing world is achievable
- Micro-credit models have exhibited a high degree of replicability
- Micro-credit programmes help borrowers work their way out of poverty
- Micro-credit programmes stimulate savings and asset accumulation among poor people
- Micro-credit programmes become vehicles for a variety of desirable social developments.

MICRO FINANCE AND POVERTY

One of the main assumptions is that many poor people can absorb, use and actively want productive credit. It is also being found that in many situations poor people want secure savings facilities and consumption loans just as much as productive credit. The poor face barriers in gaining access to formal mainstream financial service institutions. However, simple financial intermediation is not expected to be sufficient to make them participate. Micro-finance institutions (MFIs) have therefore to create mechanisms to bridge the gaps created by poverty, illiteracy, gender and remoteness. Local institutions must be built and nurtured, and the skills and confidence of new clients developed. For micro finance to succeed, some degree of social intermediation is required. Social intermediation is defined as the process of creating social capital as a support to sustainable financial intermediation with poor and disadvantaged groups or individuals. For most MFIs, social intermediation is provided through the groups or NGOs working in partnership. As Ledgerwood (1998) points out, there are four broad categories of services that may be provided:

1. Financial intermediation: It is the provision of financial products and services such as savings, credit, insurance, credit cards, and payment systems. Financial intermediation should not require ongoing subsidies.
2. Social intermediation: It is the process of building the human and social capital required by sustainable financial intermediation for the poor. Social intermediation may require subsidies for longer than financial intermediation, but eventually subsidies should be eliminated.
3. Enterprise development services: They are non-financial services that assist micro-entrepreneurs. They include: business training, marketing and technology services, skills development and sub-sector analysis. Enterprise development services may or may not require subsidies, depending on the willingness and ability of clients to pay for these services.

4. Social services: These are non-financial services that focus on improving well being of micro-entrepreneurs. They include health, nutrition, education, and literacy training. Social services will likely require ongoing subsidies, which are often provided by the state or through donors supporting NGOs".

It is assumed that the micro finance institutions by their very definition are mandated to provide financial services and intermediation. They can also offer other services as a means of improving the ability of their 'clients' to utilize financial services. For an MFI there are then, two approaches, the minimalist that sees credit as a missing piece, and the integrated, whereby all four kinds of services are provided.

In the present context we are looking at a situation whereby all the services are to be facilitated by the self-help promoting institution. It may utilize the services of the MFIs for financial intermediation and provide the social and other intermediation through its own efforts or through convergence of services etc. Group social intermediation is defined as building the institutional capacity of groups and investing in the human resources of their members so that groups can begin to function on their own with less help from outside.

CREDIT DELIVERY AND SELF HELP GROUPS (SHGs)

SHGs are now being viewed as dependable vehicles for rural credit delivery. SHGs have a number of advantages over the traditional system. In the traditional banking system, there has been a strong focus on issues like economical feasibility and loan size, collateral and guarantees, productiveness of a loan, structured loans, unit costs, scheduled assets, strict schedule for recovery, recovery rates, etc. The transaction costs are also high due to (*a*) inflexible lending terms not geared to the customers' needs, (*b*) poor monitoring due to absence of marketing information (*c*) high default rate due to political interventions, (*d*) high documentation/procedural costs for borrowers and (*e*) lack of market orientation and proper treatment (Karmakar, 1999). The system does not cater to the specific dynamics of the credit needs of the poor. The banks need to cater to the following issues:

a. Credit needs of the poor are small, emergent, and frequent. Existing systems do not allow for meeting such needs;
b. The dividing line between production and consumption loans is very thin; and
c. The poor need easily accessible credit at their doorstep.

The SHGs offer a unique opportunity for dispensing cheap credit (complementing the existing banking system) at the doorstep of the poor with almost assured repayment at the terms and requirements of the poor. The SHGs follow collective decision making on issues like meetings, thrift and credit decisions. The participative nature of the group makes it a responsible borrower. However, the most critical factor which stands out, is the fact that lending through SHGs focuses exclusively on the poor, who have hitherto been circumvented by the formal system. They initiate an empowerment process amongst the poor, specially the women.

After initial hesitation, the formal financial sector is now opening up to financing SHGs with their own operations. Linking SHGs with banks has been shown to be cost effective, transparent, and a flexible approach to improve the accessibility of credit from the formal banking system to the unreached rural poor. The provision of credit through SHGs reduces the direct transaction costs of the banks by 40–60% as a major task of appraisal, supervision, and recovery of loan is taken care of by the group itself. The transaction costs to the banks are reduced from 34% to 11% when lending to SHGs (Puhazhendhi, 1994). In addition, there is also an overall reduction in the borrower's transaction costs by approximately 85%.

Micro-credit has been advocated as the new panacea for reduction of poverty. Its potential for economic empowerment of women has also been variously looked at. Diverse groups have taken strict and distinct positions. Goetze and Gupta (1996) have questioned the naivety of the assumption that economic empowerment is a straightforward process, and easing women's access to credit translates unproblematically into their control over its use. Gopalan (2001) however cautions against dismissing micro-credit and self help groups off-hand. She reiterates that there is need to recognize the plurality in micro-credit (with savings and credit or SHGs) on one hand and extends to credit for empowerment approaches. However, given all the criticism over loan use and control and access issues, micro-credit has undoubtedly emerged as one of the entry points in engaging self-help groups of poor women in a dialogical relationship.

CREDIT FOR EMPOWERMENT

Besides being vehicles for the delivery of micro-credit, self-help groups can also be used to foster solidarity and collectivism among the rural poor, particularly the women. The SHGs can be tools to bring about holistic empowerment of the poor rural women. However, solidarity may be an expensive input for financial services production as the costs of group formation and interaction outweigh the benefits of high repayment with group control (Reinke, 1998).

Credit for empowerment is about meeting daily consumption needs of the poorest. It entails trying to build capacities of a large number of individuals, usually collectives, to increase credit absorption and undertake sustainable livelihoods. The SHG is conceived as a sustainable people's institution, which provides the poor with the space and support necessary for them to take effective steps towards achieving greater control of their lives in society. The focus is on mobilizing the poor to pool their own funds, building their capacities, and empowering them to leverage external credit.

Group formation is seen as crucial to the empowerment process as women draw strength from numbers. The group provides:

(*a*) Confidence and mutual support for women striving for social change.

(*b*) A forum in which women can critically analyse their situations and devise collective strategies to overcome their difficulties.

(*c*) A framework for awareness raising, confidence building, dissemination of information and delivery of services, and for developing communal self-reliance and collective action.

(*d*) A vehicle for the promotion of economic activities.

The 'Credit For Empowerment' strategy extends itself beyond the limited objectives of ensuring access to credit only (Gopalan, 2001). It combines the goals of financial sustainability with that of creating community-owned institutions. There have been many examples and experiences available in the country (*Swayam Shikshan Prayog*, Tamil Nadu Corporation for the Development of Women, *Swa-Shakti, etc.*), which reveal that women are empowered when savings, credit and enterprise are used as tools for mobilizing and building capacities of grassroot women collectives. They are able to acquire confidence to renegotiate gender relations, albeit to a very modest degree both within the household as well as in the larger community.

As discussed earlier, the banks find it easier to dispense credit through SHGs. The SHGs, on the other hand, are able to cater to the immediate and often emergent credit needs of the individual members. The members have the freedom, probably for the first time in their lives, to decide as to which members' credit needs are more emergent, what should be the interest rate, under what terms and conditions the loan should be dispensed, etc. This helps them to acquire confidence to manage credit, use problem-solving skills, prioritise needs, and function in a democratic manner.

The SHGs also ensure that women emerge from being passive recipients of doles to active participants and actors in decisions concerning their own lives. Women pool their expertise and create a sense of ownership in their own collective. This also gives them confidence to act as an alternate social mechanism at the grassroots. Women begin to increasingly take charge of their own local development and local governance. The group becomes, probably the first organized (though initially informal) space for poor, marginalized women to share and voice their concerns.

Savings and credit groups also provide a base for poor women to organize themselves, expand options for livelihoods and to participate actively in development. Importantly, the capacity of women is built up in spheres that were previously not their domain, for example, opening and operating bank accounts, visiting local offices, accessing loans, etc. This also presupposes a number of skills that women must acquire to be able to operate effectively in the SHG. The SHG thus often provides a platform for women to become functionally literate, sharpen communication and conflict resolution skills, and acquire skills in democratic functioning and institution building.

CONCEPT AND CHARACTERISTICS OF RURAL WOMEN SELF-HELP GROUPS

SHGs of women have been in existence for quite sometime, albeit in different *avatars*. As pointed out earlier, it is only recently, with the recognition of the Grameen model and the work of Myrada and TNWDC that they have come to acquire a prominent place in development discourse in India. Opinions on these self-help groups range from extreme skepticism (conspiracy of the capitalists to atone for the ill-effects of liberalization-globalization) to extreme optimism (ultimate panacea for all ills). However, their utility and relevance in addressing women's concerns cannot be over-emphasised.

SHGs of women have existed in India for quite sometime. Documented evidence on their exact origins may not be available. They have, however been used for a wide range of developmental goals, from service delivery to empowerment. An assortment of inputs has also been delivered through the SHGs; education and awareness generation (*Mahila Samakhya,* Rajasthan Women's Development Project); convergence of services of the line departments (Urban Basic Services Project); agriculture (Women in Agriculture Project), health services (*Mahila Swasthya Sangh*); micro-credit delivery (*Rashtriya Mahila Kosh*, NABARD, CARE, etc.); microcredit delivery and micro-enterprise development (Tamil Nadu Women's Development Project and Maharashtra Rural Credit Programme); and women's empowerment (*Swa-Shakti Project*). The much maligned and massive Integrated Rural Development Programme (IRDP) in its transformed *avatar*, the *Swarnjayanti Gram Swa-Rozgar Yojana* (SGSY), also follows the SHG mode. This apart, a number of state governments are also joining the cause. Ambitious schemes of forming SHGs in each village (Karnataka, MP, etc.) through untrained, albeit sometimes half-trained, reluctant, and disinclined functionaries of development programmes like the ICDS have been floated. Some states, like Madhya Pradesh have even established full-fledged directorates for Self-Help Groups. At the village level, we have now a situation whereby groups of women are involved in all kinds of activities ranging from watershed conservation and maintenance, primary education, health, water-use, aforestation, lands reclamation, etc. A large number of NGOs are also forming self-help groups of women for numerous reasons. Thus in my view, it is important, for development professionals to appreciate the concept and functioning of self-help groups.

SHGs, Micro finance and Empowerment are linked to each other. Empowerment is the process of acquiring the ability to make strategic life choices. Women themselves can only drive the process of empowerment; however education, capacity building, political mobilization can facilitate it, changes in systems of property rights and the social and legal institutions that marginalize women. Empowerment entails that women acquire a critical awareness of themselves as women with gendered structures of power (gender awareness), self-esteem and self-confidence (a potential for action, the ability to define one's goal and act upon them, as also feeling capable of acting upon one's goals).

It is widely assumed that micro-finance will have a positive impact on women's livelihood in the following ways:

- Leading to higher income that will help women to better perform their reproductive role as brokers of health, nutritional, and educational status of other household members.
- Increasing women's employment in micro enterprises

and in improving the productivity of women's income-generating activities.

- Enhancing their self-confidence and status within the family as independent producers and providers of valuable cash resources to the household economy. An analysis by Hashemi et al. (1996) establishes that a woman contributing to her household's income is a significant contributing factor towards her empowerment.
- It is also seen that the probability of empowerment is eight to twelve times as high for a woman who is contributing to family support or involved in a credit programme (and not contributing).
- This basically establishes that credit programmes can empower women, whether they contribute or not to family income. Participation in credit programmes per se, contributes in an independent manner to empowerment.
- A study from Bangladesh confirms improvements in women's physical mobility, economic security, ability to make own purchases, freedom from family domination and violence, political and legal awareness and public participation, as a result of a more stable integration into microfinance circuits (Schuler and Hashemi, 1994).
- A study of Grameen Bank suggests that women participants in credit programmes are more conscious of their rights, better able to resolve conflicts, and have more control over decision making at the household and community levels (Chen, 1992).
- Credit to women has positive effects on the schooling of girls; it increases women's asset holdings (except land) and is a significant determinant of total household expenditure (Pitt and Khandker, 1998).
- A study in Sri Lanka found that loans contributed to women's independent income, giving them more bargaining power in their relation with male family members (Hulme and Mosley, 1996).

- Enhanced women's empowerment, such as increased self-confidence, and better cooperation with neighbours has also been observed in Thailand (MkNelly and Watetip, 1993).
- About 63% of women's loans are actually invested by male relatives, while women bear the formal responsibility for repayment in a Bangladesh programme (Goetze and Gupta, 1996).
- A study of 151 Grameen Bank loans to women found that 12% surrendered the entire loan to male family members.
- Another study in Bangladesh discovered that of 140 loans made by ACTIONAID to women, about 50% were used for men's productive activities.
- A survey of loans to women borrowers in the Grameen Bank, Save the Children Fund and BRAC registered a loss of direct control over loan use (Ackerly, 1995).
- An assessment of K-REP confirmed that men try to control income from women's enterprises.

According to a more recent study of women borrowers in the Grameen Bank, 10 of 40 women in the sample were passing on all or most of their loans to male family members under circumstances that gave them little control over the use of this capital. On the other hand, the loss of control over financial resources does not necessarily mean that women are worse off in terms of increased social and economic opportunities (Goetze and Gupta, 1996; Todd, 1996):

- Even when women lose control over the use of their loans, their overall status in the household may improve due to their role as a financial mediator.
- Handing over loans to men may help to secure family stability by easing cashflow bottlenecks in the household.
- Women may also use credit as a bargaining chip to gain access to other opportunities offered by financial institutions, such as training, education and information (www-esd.worldbank.org/sbp/end/ngo.htm).

The impact of micro-finance services is higher when women actually control the financial resources acquired in their name. Increased control (Ackerly, 1995) is likely to contribute to women's empowerment; facilitate women's entrepreneurship; assist women in their reproductive tasks; and to ease their repayment burden.

The Government of India has been initiating some measures for the creation of models in the area of micro-credit and women's empowerment, through its programmes like the *Indira Mahila Yojana*, the *Swa-Shakti*, and the Integrated Women's Empowerment Project (*SwayamSidha*). It has also tried to create a conducive environment through the establishment of the National Credit Fund for Women (*Rashtriya Mahila Kosh*) and capacity building of field-level personnel through the distance education programme in collaboration with the IGNOU. The experience though encouraging has not been complemented with the required upscaling. The National Policy for the Empowerment of Women, adopted in April 2001, has listed a number of policy prescriptions. It is mentioned under 'Economic Empowerment of Women, 5.2 ', that " in order to enhance women's access to credit for consumption and production, the establishment of new, and strengthening of existing micro-credit mechanisms and micro-finance institutions will be undertaken so that the outreach of credit is enhanced. Other supportive measures would be taken to ensure adequate flow of credit through extant financial institutions and banks, so that all women below poverty line have easy access to credit".

The Report of the Working Group on Empowerment of Women for the Tenth Five-Year Plan (2002–07, adopted in May 2001) has pointed out that "in order to enhance women's access to credit for consumption and production, the micro-credit institutions in the country should be further strengthened and the actual flow of funds should be substantially enhanced so that self-employed groups of women have access to adequate credit for the income generating activities". In addition, it is also stated that "self-help groups of women have been found to be very effective grassroot institutions in facilitating access of women to means of development, be it information, financial and material resources or services. This mode should be encouraged, so that the groups become dynamic change agents bringing about empowerment and socio-economic development of women". However, micro-credit appears under economic empowerment diluting the social and personal empowerment, potential of micro-credit.

Similarly, in the National Policy for the Empowerment of Women, 2001, micro-credit appears under the same section on economic empowerment of women. The policy states, "In order to enhance women's access to credit for consumption and production, the establishment of new, and strengthening of existing micro-credit mechanisms and micro-finance institution will be undertaken so that the outreach of credit is enhanced. Other supportive measures would be taken to ensure adequate flow of credit through extant financial institutions and banks, so that all women below poverty line have easy access to credit"(Sec 5.2). The Plan of Action of the National Policy for the Empowerment of Women, 2001 puts forward the following steps to be undertaken in order to operationalise Section 5.2 of the policy:

a. Allocations in the coming years must address the large unmet demand for micro-finance (studies reflect large gaps between coverage and overall requirement for micro-finance), with appropriate supportive mechanism to enable long term self-employment;

b. Simplify procedures so that more women can access credit;

c. Strengthen network of institutions who provide credit so that outreach of credit can be enhanced; and

d. Build a stronger and wider network of women's micro-finance groups, so as to empower them further.

As mentioned earlier, the Government has been aggressively pursuing the concept of self-help groups at almost all levels. However, in this pursuit, a number of quality issues, especially those concerning the process of selection of the poorest of the poor, process of group formation, moving at the pace of the women, capacity-building requirements and their related quality issues, as well as rushed promotion of enterprises are some of the concerned areas that need immediate attention. In addition, what is more important is that self-help initiatives need to be encouraged and not instrumentalised into governmental initiatives. The dynamism of self-help is often eroded when put into a structured programme. Enabling conditions at all levels have to be created to facilitate the dynamism, fortitude and vitality of self-help.

REFERENCES

Ackerly, B.A. (1995). "Testing the tools of development: credit programmes, loan involvement and women's empowerment" in "Getting Institutions Right for Women in Development", *IDS Bulletin*, 26 (3).

Chen, M.A. (1992). Beyond Credit: A Subsector Approach to Promoting Women's Enterprises, Ottawa: Aga Khan Foundation.

Karmakar, K.G. (1999). *Rural Credit and Self Help Groups*. New Delhi : Sage.

King, E.M. and Andrew, M.D. (2001). Engendering Development Through Gender Equality in *Development Outreach*, 3, (2) Spring World Bank Institute.

Goetze, A.M. and Gupta, R.S. (1996). "Who Takes the Credit? Gender, Power and Control Over Loan Use in Rural Credit Programes in Bangladesh". *World Development*, 24 (1).

Gopalan, P. (2001). "The Many Faces of Micro-Credit". *Humanscape*, (August).

Government of India, Ministry of Human Resource Development Department of Women and Child Development. (2001). National Policy for Empowerment of Women, New Delhi.

Hashemi, S.S. and Riley, S. (1996). "Rural Credit Programmes and Women's Empowerment in Bangladesh", *World Development*, 24 (4).

Hulme, D. and Mosley, P. (1996). *Finance Against Poverty*. London: Routledge.

Ledgerwood, J. (1998). *Sustainable Banking with the Poor*, Washington D.C. : World Bank.

Mcguire, P.B. and Conroy, J.D. (2000). The Microfinance Phenomenon. *Asia Pacific Review*. 7, (1).

Microcredit Summit. (1997). *Declaration and Plan of Action.*

MkNelly, B. and Watetip, C.H. (1993). *Impact evaluation of Freedom from Hunger's credit with education program in Thailand.* Davis quoted in women in the informal sector and their access to microfinance IPU Annual Conference, 1998, www.gdrc.org/icm/wind/uis-wind.html.

Pitt, M. and Khandker, S. (1998). "The Impact of Group Based Credit Programmes on Poor Households in Bangladesh: Does the Gender of The Participant Matter". *Journal of Political Economy,* 106 : 958–96.

Puhazhendhi V. (1994). "Transaction Costs of Lending to the Rural Poor". Foundation for Development Cooperation and NABARD.

Reinke, J. (1998). "Does Solidarity Pay?" *Development and Change,* 29, (3).

Schuler, S.R. and Hashemi, S.M. (1994). "Credit Programs, Women's Empowerment, and Contraceptive Use in Rural Bangladesh". *Studies in Family Planning,* 25 (2) : 65–76.

Sen, K.M. and Shiva Kumar, A.K. (2001). *Women in India, How Free? How Equal*? New Delhi : Office of the United Nations Resident Coordinator in India.

Todd, H. (1996). *Women at the Center. Grameen Bank borrowers after one decade,* Oxford : Westview Press.

Venkateswaran, S. (1992). *Living on the Edge: Women, Environment and Development.* New Delhi : Friedrich Ebert Stiftung.

wcd.nic.in

World Bank. (1991). *A World Bank Country Report: Gender and Poverty in India,* Washington D.C.: World Bank.

www-esd.worldbank.org/sbp/end/ngo.htm

www.fao.org

Chapter 4

Gender Budgeting and Auditing: Insights from the Indian Experience

Adarsh Sharma

Women, who constitute half of the population, are generally not treated as equal with men in the matter of self-development although their betterment and well being are crucial to the progress, prosperity and peaceful existence of mankind. Development is meant to widen opportunities for all people. Continuing exclusion of women from many opportunities of life substantially negates the process of development.

Mainstreaming has been widely adopted as a strategy for attaining the goal of gender equality. In the 1970s and 1980s, advocates of women development talked of integrating women into development, in the 1990s the emphasis changed to the institutionalization of gender issues in development policy and planning (Goetze, 1995). Mainstreaming gender is a technical, as well as a social and political process. It requires changes at different levels such as in agenda setting, policy making, planning, budgeting practices, and resource allocations.

Gender mainstreaming in programme budget process brings gender perspective explicitly to the fore by making it an integral part of planning and decision-making processes. The Fourth World Conference of Women held in Beijing in September 1995 and the subsequent Platform for Action emphasized a gender perspective in all macro-economic policies. The twenty-third special session of the General Assembly in June 2000 also explicitly called for attention to the goal of gender equality in budgetary processes at national, regional and international levels (A/S-23/10/Reb.1, Para 65). The outcome document of the UN General Assembly urged all the nations to integrate a gender perspective into key macro-economic and social development policies. The Sixth Conference of Commonwealth Ministers of Women's Affairs held in New Delhi in April, 2000 also made similar recommendations.

> *"The realization and the achievement of the goals of gender equality, development and peace need to be supported by the allocation of necessary human, financial and material resources for specific and targeted activities to ensure gender equality at the local, national, regional and international levels as well as by enhanced and increased international cooperation. Explicit attention to these goals in the budgetary processes at the national, regional and international levels is essential."*
>
> (Twenty-third Special Session of the General Assembly to follow up implementation of the Platform for Action, June 2000 (A/S-23/10/Rev.1).

The Context

Financial and human resources have generally been insufficient universally for the advancement of women and effective implementation of the recommendations made both at the Beijing Platform for Action, and other United Nations' Summits and Conferences. The fulfilment of these obligations requires a political commitment to make available human and financial resources for the empowerment of women. Needless to emphasize that unless resources are allocated adequately and spent optimally, there can be no incremental change in the lives of women.

National budgets reflect how governments mobilize and allocate public resources, and how they aim to meet the social and economic needs of their people. Gender budgeting is a strategy for ensuring gender-sensitive resource allocation and a tool for engendering macro-economic policy. It enables tracking and allocating resources for women empowerment. It is noteworthy that national budgets may appear to be gender-neutral policy instruments, but these deal with financial aggregate—expenditures and revenues, surpluses of deficits—rather than with people. It should not be assumed therefore, that government expenditures and revenues would impact equally on men and women.

Gender Budgeting

Since the mid 1980s attempts have been made to integrate gender perspectives into national budgets. Initially the initiatives were called women's budgets; later these were called gender budgets to reflect the ongoing shift from a focus on women to the focus on gender and the relations between women and men. Another commonly used term is gender-sensitive budgets. Recently, there has been a broader use of the term mainstreaming gender perspectives into national budgets, which seems a more appropriate term since the objective is not to produce a separate gender budget but to incorporate relevant gender perspectives into national budget processes. Gendering the budget is not meant to bargain for a larger share of the resources for women or to create a separate budget for them. The aim is to analyze the budgetary expenditures from a gender perspective (Menon, 2002).

Gender Budget initiative is a methodology and set of tools and processes designed to facilitate the application of gender analysis in the formulation of government budgets and the allocation of budgetary resources. The objective is to enhance formulation of fiscal policy and measures by providing a mechanism for ascertaining their impacts on women, men, girls and boys. The initiative is neither a separate budget, nor a strategy to deliberately increase government spending on social programmes, but an instrument to enhance efficiency in utilizing and targeting available budgetary resources for the construction of a fairer and equitable society.

It involves analysis of any form of public expenditure, or method of raising revenues from a gender perspective. It includes analysis of gender-targeted allocations (e.g. special programmes targeting women); disaggregated by gender, the impact of mainstream expenditures across all sectors, services and a review of equal opportunities, policies and allocations within government services. Gender extensive budget initiatives can highlight the gaps between policy statements and the resources committed for their implementation, ensuring that public money is raised and spent in more gender equitable ways (see Figure 4.1).

Figure 4.1 : Scope of Gender Audit

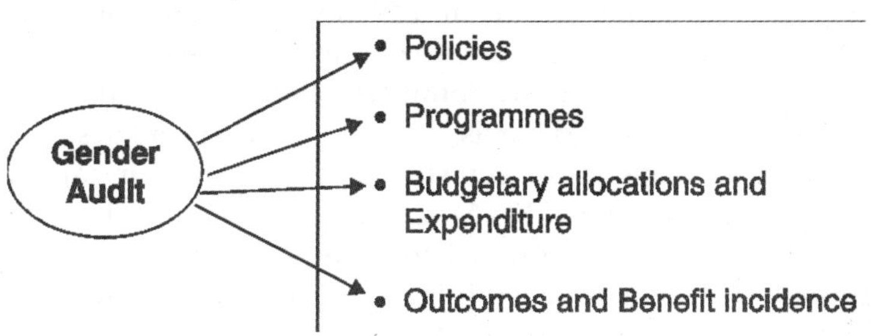

Few government revenue-raising activities or expenditures are designed on the basis of gender. Indeed, many countries have been replacing measures that were regarded as discriminatory with gender-neutral approaches (Himmelweit, 1998a: 6). For example, mother's benefits have been replaced by child allowance paid to the person who is the primary caretaker of the child. However, the goal of removing discrimination or achieving 'gender neutrality' should not be confused with the fact that budgetary policies can have significantly different impacts on women and men and on different groups of women and men. Sometimes these differences can be justified to achieve certain policy goals and sometimes they can undermine social and economic objectives. It may be mentioned that to ignore the gendered impact of policy does not constitute gender neutrality; rather, it describes 'gender blindness' (Budlender and Sharp, 1998).

Gender Budgeting: Global Scenario

Australia was the first country to develop a gender-sensitive budget, with the Federal Government publishing in 1984, the first comprehensive audit of the government budget to assess its impact on women and girls. Women's budget exercises were also undertaken by each of the Australian State and Territory Governments between the 1980s and 1990s. The Philippines was one of the few countries that began mainstreaming gender in the planning process as early as 1986. However, the gender and development budget policy was formally adopted in 1995.

South Africa also initiated the formation of a Gender-Sensitive Budget in 1995, through a participatory process of involving parliamentarians and NGOs. The commonwealth initiative to integrate gender into national budgetary processes was started in 1977 in few countries other than South Africa such as Fiji, St Kitts and Nevis, Barbados and Sri Lanka; several other nations have also taken steps to engender their national budget (Canada, the U.K., Mozambique, Namibia, Tanzania and Uganda). Gender budget initiatives are currently being attempted in 35 countries following diverse trajectories in terms of the process and partners involved in undertaking the activity.

Gender-responsive budget initiatives, either inside government or by groups within the community, on any significant scale in the world, are relatively new phenomena. In practice, gender-responsive budgets have sought to: raise awareness and understanding of the gender issues and impacts of budgets and policies; make governments accountable for their budgetary and policy commitments to gender equality; and bring about changes in budgets and policies (Sharp, 1999).

Gender Budgeting in India: Milestones

In India, the gender perspective on public expenditure had been gaining ground since the publication of the report of the Committee on the Status of Women in 1974. The need for focusing on women's issues as an exclusive subject was felt as early as in the Seventh Plan when a separate Department of Women and Child Development was created in the year 1985 and 27 women specific schemes were identified for monitoring by the Prime Minister's Office through this Department. The

Eighth Five-Year Plan (1992–97) highlighted for the first time the need to ensure a definite flow of funds from the general developmental sectors to that of women. The plan document made an express statement that "...the benefits of development from different sectors should not bypass women and special programmes on women should complement the general development programmes. The latter, in turn, should reflect greater gender sensitivity." This approach, however, could not make much dent in ensuring adequate flow of funds and benefits to women.

The Ninth Five-Year Plan (1997–2002), while re-affirming the earlier commitment adopted Women Component Plan as one of the major strategies and directed both the Central and the State Governments to ensure "...not less than 30 per cent of the funds/benefits are earmarked in all the women's related sectors." It also directed that a special vigil be kept on the flow of the earmarked funds/benefits through an effective mechanism to ensure that the proposed strategy brings forth a holistic approach towards empowering women.

The Finance Minister in his budget speech 2000 made a special reference that the year 2001 would be observed as a Women Empowerment Year. The announcement was made in the context of an urgent need for improving the access of women to national resources and for ensuring their rightful place in the mainstream of economic activity. The operational strategies outlined in the National Policy for Empowerment of Women 2001 also envisaged introduction of a gender perspective in the budgeting process.

> *"...in order to support better planning and programme formulation and adequate allocation of resources, Gender Development Indices (GDI) will be developed by networking with specialized agencies. Gender auditing and development of evaluation mechanisms will also be undertaken along side. Collection of gender disaggregated data by all primary data collecting agencies of the Central and State Governments as well as research and academic institutions in the Public and Private Sectors will be undertaken. Data and information gaps in vital areas reflecting the status of women will be sought to be filled in by these immediately. All Ministries/Corporations/Banks and financial institutions etc. will be advised to collect, collate, disseminate data*

related to programmes and benefits on a gender disaggregated basis. This will help in meaningful planning and evaluation of policies".
(National Policy for Empowerment of Women 2001– p.16).

In pursuance of the above, the Tenth Plan reinforces commitment to gender budgeting to establish its gender-differential impact and to translate gender commitments into budgetary commitments. Therefore, the Tenth Plan initiates immediate action in tying up these two effective concepts of Women Component Plan (WCP) and Gender Budgeting to play a complementary role to each other, and thus ensures both preventive and post-facto action in enabling women to receive their rightful share from all the women-related general development sectors.

Initiatives by Department of Women and Child Development

The Department of Women and Child Development, Government of India has a mandate to monitor the actions taken by different government agencies for the promotion of gender equality. In pursuance, the Department has taken several initiatives in the recent years to advocate gender sensitivity in planning and budgeting. One of the major constraints in the gender analysis of public expenditure is the non-availability of gender-disaggregated data at the state and district levels. The Department in 1998 took the initiative of generating such a data across the country to promote gender sensitivity. A series of consultations was held with States and Union Territory Administrations to develop Gender Development Index (GDI) and Gender Empowerment Measures (GEM).

The Department initiated consultations with states and union territory administrations through a workshop on Gender Issues and Indicators for States and Districts on 6–7 November 1998 followed by a workshop on developing Gender Development Index (GDI) and Gender Empowerment Measures (GEM) and establishing indicators for states and districts on 2–3 December 1998 to disseminate the concept and initiate exercises in gender-sensitive planning. Eighteen important indicators were identified for collection of gender-disaggregated data by states and districts. In July 2000, a workshop on Engendering National Budgets in the South Asian Region was organized in collaboration with UNIFEM. The Department subsequently commissioned the National Institute of Public Finance and Policy (NIPFP), New Delhi to undertake a study on gender-related economic policy issues, to cover:

- Parameters to identify status of women;
- Quantification of contribution of women;
- Assessing impact of government budget on women;
- Role women can play in improving institutional framework for delivery of public services.

Based on the interim report of the NIPFP, (January 2001), for the first time, the Economic Survey 2000–2001 highlighted issues like gender inequality and status of women. Thus gender equality and empowerment of women have been recognized as economic goals. It is to be continued as a regular feature every year. The second interim report of the NIPFP (August 2001), analyzed the Union Budget 2001–2002 from a gender perspective. Follow-up workshops on 3–4 October 2001 and 6 December 2001 were organized, culminating in initiation of measures to undertake analysis of state budgets through a network of research institutions and gender experts, under the coordination of (NIPCCD), broadly adopting the methodology of the NIPFP report on the Union Budget. Government of India has asked all ministries and departments to devote a chapter on gender issues in their annual reports, reflecting new initiatives/policies on gender-related issues, resources available and their utilization and gender disaggregated statistics, for promoting gender awareness within and outside the government.

Gender Analysis of Budget

Union Budget 2002–2003

The Department undertook analysis of the Union Budget of 2002–03 from a gender perspective, in terms of 'Pro-Women' and 'Women Specific' schemes utilizing the methodology adopted by the National Institute of Public Finance and Policy.

(*a*) Women-specific schemes are those specifically targeted at women and girls.

(*b*) Pro-women schemes have a significant women component (Table 4.1).

Table 4.1 : Summary Finding—Union Budget

Schemes	*Budget Estimates (Rs. in Crore)*		
	2001–2002	*2002–2003*	*2003–2004*
Women Specific	3260	3358	3675
Percentage variation		3%	9%
Pro Women Allocation	10596	13036	13297
Percentage variation		23%	2%

The analysis concluded that:

- Allocation on women-specific schemes increased from Rs. 3,260 crore in 2001–2002 to Rs. 3,358 crore in the Budget for 2002–2003, an improvement of three per cent.
- Allocations on most of the women-specific schemes had been enhanced. The only scheme where allocation has been reduced is the Reproductive and Child Health Programme of the Department of Family Welfare, which is attributable to the revamping of the scheme due to which some of the components of the programme are now covered under the Immunization Programme. Two schemes have been transferred to the states (*Balika Samridhi Yojana,* Post-Partum Programmes) and a few schemes have been dropped (*Mahila Samridhi Yojana,* Socio-Economic Programme, Women's Empowerment Year). Budgetary allocations on Pro-women schemes has increased from Rs. 10,596.37 crore in 2001–2002 to Rs. 13,0361.01 crore in 2002–2003, reflecting a percentage increase of 23.

Union Budget 2003–2004

An extension of this methodology has been carried out to the Union Budget of 2003–2004. The schemes have been reviewed under categories 'Women-specific Schemes' and 'Pro-women Schemes' (Table 4.1). The analysis reveals:

Women-specific Schemes

- The provision under Revised Estimates in 2002–2003 for Women-specific Schemes was Rs. 2852.61 crore as compared with Rs. 3358.21 crore provided in the Budget Estimates for 2002–2003, reflecting a reduction of 15 per cent.
- Allocation of resources for 'Women-Specific Schemes' in the Union Budget 2003–2004 stands at Rs. 3,675.37 crore reflecting an increase of 9 per cent as compared with the Budget Estimates for 2002–2003, and an increase of 29 per cent as compared with the Revised Estimates.

Pro-women Schemes

- Total budget provision in 2003–2004 for schemes identified as Pro Women, reflects an increase of 7 per cent as compared with the Budget Estimates of the previous financial year.
- The Pro Women allocation of Rs. 13297 in these schemes reflects an increase of 2 per cent.

Analysis of State Budgets

After extensive consultations with gender experts and research institutions, the Department initiated an exercise for State Gender Budget Analysis under the coordination of the NIPCCD. Gender budget studies have been commissioned for 25 states through 19 social research scientists and research organizations. The intention is to obtain a comprehensive position on the impact of public expenditure for women. Further, it would provide an analysis of the changing status of women in the selected states. The exercise covers the years: 2000–2001, 2001–2002 and 2002–2003.

Overview of the Methodology

The framework for undertaking State Gender Budget analysis

is a simple methodology of a desk review comprising scanning state budget documents to collect requisite information on the following categories of schemes and programmes:

- **Women-Targeted/Specific Schemes** defined as schemes where 100% of allocation was meant for women.
- **Pro-Women Schemes** defined as those which incorporate at least 30% of allocation for women or significantly benefit women.
- **Gender-Neutral Schemes** meant for the community as a whole.

These programmes have been further classified in four clusters on the basis of their potential impact on women's social position and social equality. The four categories are:

- **Protective services**, such as allocations on women's homes and care institution, rehabilitation schemes for victims of atrocities, pensions for widows and destitute women, etc. which are aimed at directly benefiting the women mitigating the consequences of women's social and economic subordination, rather than addressing the root causes of this subordination.
- **Social services** such as schemes for education and health of women, support services like crèche and hostels and also water supply, sanitation and schemes on fuel and fodder, which contribute significantly to women's empowerment, either directly by building their capacities and ensuring their material well being or indirectly through reducing domestic drudgery.
- **Economic services** such as schemes for training and skills development, and provision for credit, infrastructure, marketing, etc. which are critical to women's economic independence and autonomy.
- **Regulatory services** which include institutional mechanisms for women's empowerment, such as state commissions for women, women's cells in police stations, family counselling centres, awareness generation programmes, etc. which provide institutional spaces and opportunities for women's empowerment.

Financial allocations to these identified schemes with categorization have been analyzed further for the years 2000–2001, 2001–2002 and 2002–2003 comprising:

(*a*) Scheme-wise/Sector-wise BE/RE/Actual Expenditure.
(*b*) The percentage of BE/RE/Actual Expenditure in relation to total budget in relation to total social sector budget.
(*c*) The percentage of gap between BE and RE and between RE and Actual Expenditure in both Plan and non plan in various identified schemes.
(*d*) Across departments comparisons of allocation for women's specific/targeted and Pro-Schemes (only for departments identified as woman intensive).
(*e*) Cluster-wise allocation to schemes and programmes within departments and across states.

Budgetary Allocations for Women

In the initial attempt, data could be collated from only ten states—Assam, Bihar, Meghalaya, Gujarat, Jammu and Kashmir, Maharashtra, Rajasthan, Madhya Pradesh, Orissa and Manipur. Findings on patterns in allocation of resources for women based on preliminary analysis of the state budgets of ten states revealed some interesting trends (Table 4.2, NIPCCD, etc. 2002).

Social Sector Allocations

Assam, Meghalaya and Manipur allocated a substantial percentage of the state budget to social sector. In other states, the social sector budget received around 22–36% of the State Budget allocations in 2000–2001. The variations between two temporal series were as large as 12–29% reduction in the subsequent year (Assam, Bihar and Manipur). Rajasthan, Gujarat and Meghalaya and others had shown increase in their social sector allocation during the second year arising mainly due to increased non-Plan outlays.

Allocation to Women Programmes

In ten selected states, the range of allocations to women

Table 4.2 : Gender Budget Analysis: Summary Trends for Ten States

Indicators	*Range of Percentage share*	
	2000–2001	*2001–2002*
Share of social sector in total state budget	22% to 52%	18% to 48%
Share of women-targeted schemes in social sector budget	0.6% to 10.1%	0.8% to 10.8%
Share of women-targeted and Pro-women schemes in social sector budget	7.6% to 44.3%	6.5% to 41.3%
Share of social services in women targeted schemes	68.3% to 97.6%	67.8% to 99%
Share of social services in pro-women schemes	10.4% to 91.2%	9.6% to 89.8%
Share of economic services in pro-women schemes	5.8% to 64.1%	4.6% to 65.5%

Source : NIPCCD and DWCD (2002) Gender Budget Analysis of selected states and initiative, pp. 23, 28.

programmes (targeted and pro combined) varied from 3% to 13% of the state budget. Targeted schemes as compared to pro-women schemes received lower percentage allocations and in four states it was less than 1%. Allocation to pro-women schemes showed vide variations across states and ranged from less than 1% to 11%. It is obvious that fiscal flow to women's programme in all states was far below the desired level and lower than the norms of the Planning Commission (30%).

Of the Social Sector Budget, the women component (Pro and Targeted) received low percentage allocations in Madhya Pradesh (6.5%), modest in Rajasthan, Assam, Jammu and Kashmir, Gujarat (12%–23%) and Bihar and high percentage in Orissa and Manipur (34–44%). The percentage allocations to women target programmes of the social sector budgets were less than 5% in Bihar, Madhya Pradesh, Orissa, Assam and Manipur less than 1%. The funds earmarked for pro-women schemes were around 20–25% of the social sector allocations except in Rajasthan, Jammu and Kashmir and Madhya Pradesh.

Cluster-wise Analysis

Cluster-wise analysis of schemes and programmes showed similar trends in both categories. The highest percentage was contributed by social services followed by economic services in all states. Protective and welfare services and regulatory services were non-existent, comprising negligible percentages of the cumulative total.

Allocations to different clusters reflect the sensitivity awareness and strategic approach of the state towards planning of women empowerment programmes. It is clear from the above analysis that the ten states included in the study have made an attempt to propose allocations for schemes and services in the social service cluster that directly has a bearing on the well being of women and provide support services for their development. This cluster includes allocations to programmes for education, health, supply of fuel and fodder, drinking water, etc. In theory, at least, these schemes have the potential to contribute to empowerment of women and enable them to actively participate in their own development.

The states somehow, have not been able to plan and initiate an adequate number of schemes related to Economic Services, aimed at building skills for income-generation activities, marketing, credit availability, etc. It may be pointed out that this cluster is critical for women's empowerment, economic independence and autonomy. It is, therefore, important to re-orient the policies related to women-targeted schemes and have a holistic perspective of women's development in the planning process. Similarly, planning related to Regulatory Services requires attention. Unless institutional mechanisms are created to guard against violations of the rights of women and generate awareness, the inequality in genders cannot be bridged.

LESSONS LEARNT

The study is a step forward in refining the methodology of budget analysis. The other outcome of the endeavour has been identification of gaps in maintenance of data in gender-disaggregated form in states at the levels of different departments and for schemes related to empowerment of women. Involving states at this juncture to initiate introduction of the system of gender disaggregation for performance targets and allocation of funds may go a long way in refinement of the methodology of the budget analysis in hand.

Despite limitations, the data analysed so far has revealed a plethora of possibilities for future action and research:

- Analysis can be extended to cover a longer period of time, to establish whether there is a perceptible pattern, responsive to gender demands.
- Inter state and intra state comparison warrants deeper analysis. Allocation of resources for women (direct and indirect) needs to be correlated with parameters like population, status of women in terms of nutrition, health, education, economic empowerment, security, etc.
- Quantifiable physical targets have to be generated to monitor incidence of expenditure for women and these in turn must also be correlated with accepted indicators of status of women like literacy level, MMR, etc.
- Pattern of sectoral share of different clusters of services (Protective, Social, Economic and Regulatory) in Women-Targeted and Pro-Women Schemes, when co-rrelated with status of women, can help establish causal relationships.
- Given the variations in size of states, population, differences in urbanization and industrialization, variation in resources, etc. absolute budgetary allocations would not lend themselves to any meaningful analysis. However, comparison of percentages of provision and pattern of expenditure and trend over time would certainly give a fair indication of gender sensitivity. These, when eventually linked with physical parameters on gender status, can give a fairly good gender profile of states.

ISSUES OF CONCERN

1. Capacity building is needed for generating

disaggregated data for planning, accounting and auditing at different levels.

2. Benefit incidence analysis is central to assessing the distributional impact of budgetary allocations and impact of budgetary policies. Focusing on how much money has been allocated for schemes benefiting women can be counter-productive if the outcomes of the schemes depart substantially from the objectives that they were designed to serve.
3. Budgeting allocations of resources alone hardly throw light on the impact it would have had due to significant spread between the Budget Estimation, Revised Estimation and between Revised Estimation and Actual Expenditure. It imposes major limitations as it refers only to the intentions of the planners and not to what has actually happened.
4. There is an urgency of sharpening the methodological tools for monitoring the progress of Women's Component Plan introduced in the Ninth Five-Year Plan.
5. Extend the nature and scope of gender analysis of budgets to include benefit incidence analysis in specific geographical and sectoral areas and over a larger time frame.
6. Promote capacity building of research organizations for such an analysis particularly for in-depth studies and qualitative information through micro-level studies.
7. Restrictions to be imposed on re-appropriation of budgetary allocation meant for women and girls not to be used for any other purpose. It is essential to ensure that public funds so earmarked are spent on intended purposes.
8. Availability of gender-disaggregated data is promoted in all agencies/organizations/departments.
9. Isolating women component in local-level resource allocations.
10. Reliability and validity of data be ensured through training and identifying sound database resources.

CONCLUSIONS

It can be stated at the end that the gender budget initiative can contribute directly to improving the efficiency of resource allocations and to the strengthening of economic governance through a framework that can enhance accountability and transparency. It is noteworthy that gender budgeting is not restricted to post-audit of public accounts but has to have a comprehensive approach aimed at mainstreaming of gender issues in all aspects of public life Department of Women and Child Development, 2003 (DWCD, 2003). It is heartening that India has made a beginning and has taken initiatives, which are perhaps pioneering. These can go a long way in achieving gender equality when extended to policies, programming, public expenditure outcome and benefit incidence. Needless to say, it requires to be supported by the political commitment as well.

REFERENCES

Budlender, D. and Sharp, R. (1998). How to do a gender-sensitive budget analysis: Contemporary research and practice. Canberra, Australia: AUSAid and London: Commonwealth Secretariat.

Goetze, A. (Ed). (1995). Getting institutions right for women; *IDS Bulletin*, 26 (3). Sussex, U.K: Institute of Development Studies.

Government of India, Ministry of Human Resource Development, Department of Women and Child Development. Annual Report (2000-01), New Delhi.

Government of India, Ministry of Human Resource Development, Department of Women and Child Development. (2003). India Country Paper. Taking stock of progress made and challenges ahead. Commemorating Beijing Fourth Regional Ministerial Meeting Bhutan. May 2003, New Delhi.

Government of India, Ministry of Human Resource Development, Department of Women and Child Development. (2001). National Policy for Empowerment of Women, New Delhi.

Government of India, Planning Commission. (1977). Ninth Five-Year Plan (1997-2001), New Delhi.

Government of India, Planning Commission. (2002). Tenth Five-Year Plan (2002-2007), New Delhi.

Himmelweit, S. (1998). 'Care and the budgetary process', paper presented at out of the margins: Feminist approaches to economics, a conference, Amsterdam: 2-5 June, The Netherlands: University of Amsterdam.

Lahiri, A. (2001). Gender Budgeting in India Post-budget Assessment Draft Report.

Sen, M. K. and Prabhu, K.S. (2001). The budget: A quick look through a 'gender lens'. *Economic and Political Weekly,* 14 April: 1164–1170.

Menon, N. (2002). The women factor in budget. *The Pioneer,* 15 February.

NIPCCD and DWCD. (2002). Gender budget analysis of selected States—An initiative interim report. New Delhi.

Sharp, R. (1999). Women's Budgets. In Meg Lewis and Janice Peterson (eds.), *Dictionary of Feminist Economics.* New York: Educational Elgar.

United Nations. (1996). Fourth World Conference on Women (Beijing, 4–15 September, 1995). Platform for Action and the Beijing Declaration, New York: The author.

Valdeavilla, E.V. (2001). Gender sensitive planning and budgeting: insights from Philippines experience. Paper presented at Training workshop on gender sensitive planning and budgeting (Dar Es Salaam Tanzania: 3–7 December).

Chapter 5

Women in Governance in India

Susheela Kaushik

As an ancient country, India has had the legacy of village governments and decentralised governance from time immemorial. Ancient Indian history is replete, with references to the village republics. The benign feudal kings responded to local needs, aspirations and norms and practised an accountable democracy based on people's opinion and public approval. Following invasions and foreign rule, this practice somewhat disappeared. Government from above and even beyond, became the prevalent practice especially during the British colonial rule. From the time of the Freedom Struggle, the need for popular participation in the democratic process had been accorded much importance. Gandhi and Nehru had evoked such a participation as a political weapon against the British rulers. Mahatma Gandhi, leader of the Nationalist Movement propounded a village-centred political system called *'Gram Swarajya'*. Gandhi also believed strongly in democracy at the grassroots in the form of village self-government and considered villages to be the basic political units of the future independent nation. He felt that the Centre of Power is not in Delhi or in Calcutta (now Kolkata) or in Bombay (now Mumbai) but in the seven hundred thousand villages in India.

Women in Local Governance

Since Independence, India has adopted many policies and

measures to improve the conditions of women and enhance their status in the society and the family. A variety of approaches had been adopted, depending on one's view of women's role in society and polity. To many like Gandhi and Nehru, women were the integral part of nation builders; to play that role effectively women needed to be liberated from the debiting domestic subordination and treated at par with men in the political and domestic roles. They were to be viewed not as helpless damsels in distress, but as strong-willed and opinionated, energising, guiding and leading the family and the community. They believed, along with Vivekanand and Subhash Chandra Bose that women were capable of any role, provided they are liberated from the superstition of the 'kitchen' religion of India, and their physical and mental powers given a space for display.

The contribution of women in the Freedom Struggle and the various roles they played—from the dangerous to the routine—only convinced national leaders like Gandhi and Nehru that independent India needed them to participate in politics as voters and candidates. This led to a very early attempt to remove some of the limitations in social norms and economic disabilities. Nehru, a powerful votary of the Uniform Civil Code, was forced to dilute it as the Hindu Code Act; but still managed to get a few socio-economic rights for the Hindu women. But these rights were essentially for Hindu women, while the Muslim and Christian women continued to be governed by the religious personal codes.

However, with these reforms in family laws, the government and the nation seemed to believe that they had done all that had to be done for women, and that the latter would be able to emerge into the public sphere as empowered and free individuals, and intelligent citizens. However, instead of women emerging into the helm of governance in great numbers, the impact on women was only marginal. Women continued to remain excluded from the public sphere and particularly in the political and governing process. The increase in employment and public activities was essentially at the lower levels with secondary power and positions than at the managerial and decision-making levels. Whether in administrative posts, or at the legislative, executive and judicial levels, or in the private corporate sphere, the increase in the number of women was almost invisible. It was not before 1984 that women received the necessary boost, under the Prime Ministership of Rajiv Gandhi. The State showed sensitivity to the changes taking place in the rest of the world.

A series of world conferences on women (1975, 1980, 1985 and 1995) has aided in projecting the various concerns of women at the national and international fora. Involvement of players like the government, civil societies and international supporting organizations has influenced the process of change at various levels. A definite direction and array of strategies have emerged over the past two decades. Participation of women in governance has emerged as a salient issue before the women's movement in India in the last decade. This is because the need for the presence and participation of women in higher decision-making levels in the government, political, public and private sector institutions and non-governmental organisations in effective critical numbers, has been keenly felt. Such a participation, it is strongly believed, is a pre-requisite for not merely women's access to equality and rights, for their advancement and that of society, but also for achieving the goals of development, democracy and peace in the social order. By participating in the decision-making process in a critical number, women will also be able to transform the nation's development. This would help to preserve and promote equality and justice, monitor and reverse the existing patriarchal situation and bring about the necessary policy changes and social restructuring.

An increasing number of organizations and people working for gender equality, women's development and peace in India and abroad, are getting involved in monitoring the nature and extent of women's participation in governance, as they are of the firm conclusion that women need to play a more effective role in the decision-making process and participate in formulating policies and measures for their own development.

- Their share in the Rajya Sabha (Upper House) has been marginally better with 9 per cent representation. The situation in State Assemblies is appalling, with an overall average of 4 per cent women members of legislative assemblies (MLAs) across legislatures.
- The Women's Reservation Bill continues to be blocked. It has been revived and reintroduced with each change in government. However, the very fact of it continuing to be a live issue shows that there is a broad political consensus on the need for such reservation.
- However, reservation can at best be an interim arrangement. It cannot be a substitute for a democratic process and participation of women based on their own merit, status and right to equality.
- The political parties are, by and large, reluctant to choose women as candidates, as they are viewed as depriving men of their chances. Even the small number of women who contest, gain their candidature by their relationship with already established male party leaders.
- The nature of participation of women in governance has not been spread out to all areas of decision making. It shows that those women members who have been by and large participating, are in what are familiarly called 'women's issues' such as health, welfare, sexual atrocities, social crimes like dowry, violation of women's rights, etc. Participation in debates on wider economic, defence and political issues are often scanty. By way of leadership roles, women ministers are often entrusted with only welfare-oriented portfolios like women and child development and welfare of other weaker sections. Spheres involving technical information and expertise like finance, home, defence are rarely allotted to women, even though women have demonstrated their ability even as Prime Ministers.
- These power structures continue to be dominated by men.
- Opposition by patriarchal forces to quota by political parties as well as for the parliament and employment

continues.

- The structures and values that believe in women's subordination in the family and community, and which force women to combine traditional duties with political roles, continue to obstruct women's taking on political roles.

Challenges and Obstacles

- Only recently the three major Trade Unions, INTUC, AITUC and CITU have paid some attention to women workers and their issues.
- The patriarchal attitude of the male workers and their leaders is also responsible for: (*a*) poor representation of women in the decision-making positions, and (*b*) the issues concerning women not being taken up. However, the trade unions cover mainly the organised sectors and much of women's work falls under the unorganised sector.
- On the whole, women party members have failed to push for a gender balance within their own parties. In 1997, the Communist Party of India—Marxist (CPM) had only five women in its 70-member Central Committee. The Communist Party of India (CPI) and 12 women in its 150 member National Council and only three of the 21 members of the national executive are women. However, recently the Politbureau of CPI(M) has one women as member.
- Although the BJP has been the only party to amend its constitution to ensure the participation of women, the number was restricted to only two women per committee. That this gesture was mere public posturing became clear when only eight women found a place in the BJP's 75 member working committee. In its 650–member national council, only 150 are women. In 1997, there were just two women in its 17-member all-important election committee and there are no women representatives in its equally important manifesto, disciplinary or organizational disputes committees.

- The CPI discussed the possibility of reserving posts for women within the party at the time of drafting its manifesto in 1998. But the overriding consensus was not to commit to any fixed percentage.
- Opposition by a few political parties based on religion and caste for quota for women's representation in Parliament continues. It has even succeeded in stalling the Constitutional Amendment.
- The electoral system, with its base on money power, business deals, complicated intricacies and muscle power is not conducive to women's involvement in politics.
- The political parties are divided over the Women's Reservation Bill displaying patriarchal outburst and discontent. The pressure built by women's organizations is evident on the government.
- The decentralization also remains an incomplete process. The monitoring and implementing, rather than planning and decision-making powers are being entrusted to the local bodies. Women are still to get into the centre of it all.
- Inadequate powers and paucity of resources have limited the outreach of the National Commission for Women (NCW). Their annual reports have not been discussed by Parliament or reviewed since its inception.
- Many of the NCW recommendations for legal reforms (e.g., on the right to matrimonial property, amendment to rape and dowry legislation, adoption and guardianship rights, etc.) are still to be considered by the government. Its powers and prestige seem to be based on personalities rather than the statutory powers.
- Only a small percentage of women is visible at higher levels of bureaucracy. Only four women secretaries and two women judges in the Supreme Court were seen during these five years.
- The two-children norm enacted by the states of Andhra Pradesh, Haryana, Orissa, Rajasthan and others, to

prevent candidates with more children to contest elections (as a part of the promotion of family planning and population control measures) will act as a deterrent to common women participating in the elections from panchayat to national level.

- Globalization and structural adjustment have brought down the intensity of trade union activity. The caste, cultural and political allegiances have also hampered the women's solidarity as women and as workers.

Ever since 1951 when India adopted the reservation as tool to empowerment as mechanism concept and practice of reservation as a tool to empower the weaker sections, it has emerged as a popular and efficacious way of addressing the issues of participatory democracy and distributive justice in India. It was believed that political representation and participation of the weaker sections will lead to their political empowerment and thereby to their social and economic development. By the very first Amendment to the Constitution in 1951, the state provided reservation for Scheduled Caste (SCs) and Schedule Tribe (STs). In proportion of these castes and tribes to the total population of India, seats were reserved for them in the Parliament and State Assemblies. While the emerging picture may not be too satisfactory, there can be no denying the fact that but for the quota and reservation, the SC and ST would not have made the progress that they have achieved so far.

Best Practices

The running theme in the debates on local self government from 1957 to 1989 was one of how to enable the people to participate in the government. Parallel to this, has been the women's movement which particularly focussed on making women's participation in politics and local self government meaningful and effective.

The Report of the Committee on the Status (1974), discussed at length the participation of women in politics in general, and in panchayats in particular. The National Perspective Plan for Women in 1988–2000 A.D. and the report of the National Commission on Self-Employed Women (1988), recommended that 30 per cent of the executive head-level positions should be reserved for women from the village to the district level bodies.

With the 73rd and 74th Constitutional Amendments (1993) enhancing the powers of the local self governments and enlarging the representation to include the people from the weaker sections, equality of opportunity in decision making has become accessible even to women from rural and backward areas. This has offered women of all castes, classes and regions, an immense opportunity to have a say in the decisions which affect not merely their lives but also the area in which they reside and the nation to which they belong.

It thus, heralded the ascent of nearly one million women including those from the poorer castes and classes and the tribes, to political positions in the length and breadth of India at its rural grassroots level, where the extent of patriarchy, illiteracy, poverty and socio-cultural norms are even deeper and more strangling than in the urban areas. The reservation of seats, the instrument that made it possible, is now being advocated to enable women to emerge in national and state politics too.

The quota system has been a great boon for the women, especially in rural India. It enabled more women to come forward and to contest, and assured their election to at least one-third of the total membership. Even in the cities where urbanization and modernization have enabled more women to be developed, the number of women contesting for Parliament or state legislatures or getting elected, has been a bare minimum. The mandatory provision, thereby had brought millions of women to enter the election fray, learn their tasks on hand, sustain themselves in politics if they wish to, and move upward if they can.

India has stood out as the first democracy that initiated the experiment of giving its women special provisions of quota of one-third of total membership and chairpersonship in the local self-government bodies, thereby enabling them to participate in governance and leadership roles. Such an affirmative action had been necessitated by the widely held view that the women of lower caste are not socially free or capable of exercising their political rights; that such political consciousness and the capacity to participate in the decision-making process is confined, at best, to the urban, highly educated, middle-class elite women.

Their turnout in elections and in different meetings disproves the scepticism that they are not interested in politics. The eagerness to recontest has also taken deep root in them. Over the years, with increasing political participation the panchayats members have developed affiliations with political parties/local leaders approaching them.

The elected women have, in general, shown much interest in their role as members and chairpersons. Though initially they were shy and often ignorant too, gradually many of them have begun attending the meetings regularly. In meetings and various programmes of the local governments the attendance of the women members has increased to a substantial level not only quantitatively but also qualitatively. Being aware of their sphere of action and the importance attached to it, they are now able to put forth their views and take decision on their own. Many elected women are seeking information, attending outside meetings, choosing to get themselves trained and opting to go out of the villages.

This 'revolution' is well appreciated in the context of the worldwide movement for increased participation of women in politics and decision-making, as a necessary instrument for eliminating the discrimination and violence against them. The world is now convinced that without such a sharing in the political power, the objectives of peace, equality and development for women will be hard to achieve.

A brief look at what the women have prioritised as agenda for themselves and the local governments that they are part of, is clear evidence that the women have aspired to bring about the social development of their area. Unlike the male preference for construction of buildings and roads, the women plan for women and child welfare centres, maternity clinics, schools, etc.

However, such a social development or specific women's development cannot be achieved overnight, after so many years of neglect by previous local governments and state authorities. To expect women to bring about women's empowerment and social development in a span of five years is asking too much.

The enormity of the task of reaching these goals often frustrates the women in the initial stages. They soon understand reservation alone is not enough; other support structures and services are needed. Some of them also recognise that unless they help themselves with various opportunities, political empowerment will not reach them. These women, articulate and brave, have made efforts to meet the varied challenges emanating from various sources and sustained themselves in politics and public life. They, in turn, are also accessing the various positive factors by way of legislations, training, support of NGOs, sensitized males and bureaucracy, media publicity, information and exposure, political socialization in their background, etc. The experiment in local government has thus interesting possibilities, following the emergence and participation of a critical mass of women and weaker sections.

The last few years of women's participation in local governments have proved that the local governments can prove to be the most effective and sensitive vehicle for rectifying gender imbalances and promoting women's interest. There are more and more success stories of women helping to transform the social status quo through panchayats. To some extent the women members and chairpersons have made the local bodies responsive to women's gender-related problems. The women have implemented various schemes under the Integrated Rural Development Programme (IRDP). Raising chickens and pigs are some of the income-generating schemes introduced for women. But the real achievement lies in what the women do themselves now in order to tend to their needs. "When a tube well needs repair, women get it repaired. When a well needs to be cleaned, they buy the bleaching power and clean it. They have got over the mentality of depending on the men to get the job done", said one woman chairperson.

Women can express women's concerns better. When a woman heads the panchayat, women find a place to speak. A few years ago, women in the villages had no one to turn to if they were tortured by in-laws, said a panchayat chairperson from Haryana. "Today, they come running to the women members of the local government. We go immediately, even if it is during night."

However, in performing their functions as political leaders and people's representatives, women face quite a few challenges and difficulties.

Despite the provision of reservation of one-third seats for women, the political males have not yet reconciled to them. It is this attitude which hinders the women from full-scale participation in the decision-making process. According to a woman chairperson from Tamil Nadu, "No matter how well women function in politics, they are not taken seriously. Any idea put forth by us was defeated by men, as according to them women are only best suited for domestic responsibilities."

Many women who were conscious of these difficulties mentioned lack of domestic assistance, child care facilities, transport, political information, etc. Male domination, lack of political and financial powers, role of political parties, casteism, lack of literacy, domestic responsibilities, patriarchal taboos, harassment, violence, etc. are some of the challenges which the women members face. But with time, women have increasingly become aware of their rights, their status and political participation.

Education is responsible for unfolding the capacities that are latent in an individual. It makes one aware of one's capabilities. In local governments the literate and educated women do not have as many problems as faced by their not-so literate and educated colleagues. The latter are kept in the dark either by the government officials are the other male members of the panchayat. Being educated makes them aware of the scope of their duties and responsibilities and makes them perform their duties satisfactorily. It also helps them to check corruption, monitor the work and disseminate the message. Education also makes them positive, confident and assertive and prepares them to face the obstacles and not be cowed down by challenges. According to many women, the status of women members can improve only with more literacy and education.

Still the Panchayati Raj institutions experiment has been successful in bringing out the hidden talents of women as leaders of the community. By and large, the society and males have gracefully accepted the women in politics. However, this is not universal. Obviously it will take more time, experience and support for women to emerge as leaders and sustain their influence even after they cease to be chairpersons.

Has gender been able to overcome caste and class? To a great extent, the political power has given women from lower caste and class, a higher status and women of different castes are able to work together and organise on issues. The caste women have welcomed the entry of SC women and accepted them happily as chairpersons. It may, however, be sometime before it leads to the obliteration of caste hierarchy in the wider community.

TABLE 5.1 : Women's Presence in Top Decision Making Committees

Party	*Committee*	*No. of Women*	*Total Members*	*% of Women*
CPI (M)	Politburo	0	15	0
	Central Committee	5	70	7
CPI	Secretariat	0	9	0
	National Executive	3	31	10
	National Council	*6–7	125	5
JD	Political Affairs Committee	0	15	0
	Parliamentary Board	0**	15	0
	National Executive	11	75	15
UF	Steering Committee	0	15–17***	0
BJP	Parliamentary Board	1	9	11
	Election Committee	2	17	12
Congress	Working Committee	2	19	11

* The seventh member is a candidate member who participates in discussions but does not vote.

** Normally the state President of the JD women's wing is invited to attend and offer suggestions, but she does not have a vote. Even this invitation depends upon the wishes of Party President of the Parliamentary Board.

*** Total number of members vary due to visitors.

Source: Manushi (1996) September – October 1996, p.27.

TABLE 5.2 : General Elections in India Voters' Turnout 1952–1999

Year	*Total Electorate*		*Voting Percentage*		
	Men	*Women*	*Total*	*Male*	*Female*
1952	95,268	77,946	60.50	53.00	37.10
1957	1,02,206	91,446	63.70	56.00	39.60
1962	1,13,944	1,02,428	55.00	62.10	46.60
1967	1,30,424	1,20,174	61.00	66.70	55.50
1971	1,43,475	1,30,617	55.10	69.70	49.15
1977	1,67,019	1,54,155	60.00	65.62	54.91
1980	1,85,210	1,70,380	75.90	57.69	51.29
1984	1,96,730	1,82,810	62.40	63.61	68.17
1989	—	—	62.00	70.90	43.90
1991	—	—	53.50	52.56	47.43
1996	—	—	55.00	—	—
1998	31,48,077,909	28,75,32,4773	62.04	66.06	58.02
1999	32,15,19,865	29,28,00,744	59.83		

Source: Election Commission of India Reports.

TABLE 5.3 : Percentage of women candidates to total no. of candidates fielded by five major political parties in Lok Sabha Election (All India) in 1996, 1998 and 1999.

Sl. No.	Name of the political Party	Total No. of Contestants			No. of Women Contestants			% of Women Candidates			Women Won		
		1996	1998	1999	1996	1998	1999	1996	1998	1999	1996	1998	1999
1.	Indian National Congress	540	474	453	9	31	50	9.20	6.54	11.03	16	9	14
2.	BJP	422	384	339	23	31	25	5.92	8.07	7.37	13	13	14
3.	Janata Dal	319	190	96	13	9	4	4.07	4.73	—	4	—	—
4.	CPI (M)	76	71	72	5	8	5	6.57	11	—	2	3	3
5.	CPI	43	58	54	4	6	4	9.30	26	6.94	1	1	1
6.	SP	—	165	151	3	14	12	—	10	—	2	3	—
7.	Others	—	—	—	—	96	—	—	34	6.94	1	13	15
8.	Independent	—	—	—	500	76	—	—	—	6.89	—	—	—
Total		14274	4708	4254	599	271	278	4.3	5.7	6.5	39 (7.1%)	43 (7.97%)	48 (8.9%)

Compiled by the author from Election Commission Reports.

TABLE 5.4 : Performance of National Parties

	Party	Women Contested	Candidates Won	%
1.	BJP	30	10	33.33%
2.	BSP	20	1	5.00%
3.	CPI	2	-	
4.	CPM	8	5	62.50%
5.	INC	45	12	26.67%
6.	NCP	5	2	40.00%
	National Parties: (Total 6)	110	30	27.27%
	State Parties:	67	14	20.90%
	Registered (unrecognised) Parties:	61	1	1.64%
	Independents:	117	-	
	Total:	465	75	12.68%

Source: Election Commission of India—General Elections, 2004 (14th Lok Sabha).

REFERENCES

Government of India, Ministry of Education and Social Welfare. (1974). Towards Equality: Report of the Committee on the Status of Women in India, New Delhi.

Government of India, Ministry of Human Resource Development, Department of women and Child Development. (1998). *Shram Shakti*—Report of National Commission on Self Employed Women, New Delhi.

Government of India, Ministry of Human Resource Development, Department of Women and Child Dvelopment. (1998). National Perspective Plan for Women in the Informal Sector. (1988–2000), New Delhi.

Kishwar M. (1996). Out of Zenana Dabba: Strategies for Enhancing Women's Political Representation, *Manushi,* Issue No. 96 : 21–30.

United Nations. (2000). Convention on Elimination of All Forms of Discrimination Against Women.

United Nations. (2000). Department of Public Information (2001), Platform for action and the Bejing declaration: Fourth World Conference on women 4–15 September 1995, New York.

Website: http://www.eci.gov.in/ElctionResults/Election_Results_fs.htm

Chapter 6

Education Among Muslim Women: A Situational Analysis

Hajira Kumar

Islam has always encouraged learning among its followers. In spite of this, Muslims as a community have not been able to make a mark in the educational field. If one looks at the Holy Quran, Sura Alaq, Ayat No. 1–5 and 28–35, the act of teaching and learning has been accorded a lot of importance. Similar sentiments have also been highlighted in Sura Baqr. Prophet of Islam has himself said, "Learning is a must for every Muslim man and woman." (*Ibn Majid*). He further goes on to say that parents must educate their children (*Tirmizi Sharif*). He also says that scholars are the successors of prophets (*Tirmizi Abu Dawood*). It seems that the religious verdict and Prophet's appreciation has not created impact and in practice, the Muslim community in India has been indifferent to teaching and learning. Generally education should include: (*i*) three Rs (*ii*) vocational training, and (iii) discipline and virtuous behaviour. Unfortunately, by and large, majority of Muslims are not much interested in these three dimensions of education. This is evident from recent findings, which tell us that general literacy among women in India is nearly 39% whereas Muslim women are often illiterate or half literate. It is disheartening to see that Muslim women are so deprived.

Women of early Islamic days present a picture of sharp contrast to the disempowered Indian Muslim women of today. Religious studies, medicine, trade, teaching, social service and nursing were the fields where women created history during that time. Hazrat Khatija (R.A.A.) was a businesswoman and the services of Prophet Mohammad (SAW) were hired by her. After marriage she lived with him for nearly twenty-eight years and continued to conduct her business. Hazrat Ayesha, another wife of the holy Prophet, was the source of knowledge in every field. Ahmad quotes Urwah Bin Zubairi (R.A.A.) who said about her, "Hazrat Ayesha knows more about the injunctions of Holy Quran, poetry and literature, the history of Arabs and their hierarchy than any other person" (Ahmad, 2003 : 101). She had knowledge about medicine, accounts and legal matters as well. All the Prophet's companions were always willing to help the needy and deprived people especially the women, who were also very active. Besides, almost all the wives of the nobles used to accompany them as nurses in the battlefield where they used to work as suppliers and controllers of essential commodities. When we compare this situation with the contemporary lifestyle of Indian Muslim women, we see a lot of difference. We find a marginalized, segregated and disempowered (economically, socially and politically) group, which is characterized by a low self-profile whereas in early Islamic days women were even issuing religious verdicts (Fatwas). Some women who have left a mark are Hazrat Ayesha, Hazrat Umme Salma, Hazrat Hafza, Hazrat Jawairia, Hazrat Maimoona, Hazrat Fatima Bin Qais, to name a few.

It is very difficult to find out as to who is responsible for this situation. Is it too much and self-styled religiosity or is it mistrust and fear syndrome of a minority community which makes them feel that they should keep away from the mainstream scientific or vocational education?

Both these interpretations may not be fully correct. Muslim women were educated, knowledgeable and well respected during the early days in Islamic history. As pointed out earlier, many women during that period were recognized scholars and even issued Fatwas. Besides others, it shows that Islamic traditions support teaching, learning and educational activities among women and the view that religiosity hinders learning is not correct. As far as minority syndrome and less confident attitude is concerned, that is also not logical because Muslims are adjusted to the Indian ethos since so many centuries. Although communal riots try to break it, composite culture exists even today to a great extent. The tradition of illiteracy among Indian Muslims is in fact due to the migration of the Muslim middle class to Pakistan. Most of the Muslims who migrated to Pakistan were educated, opinionated, and politically conscious people and those who remained at their native places were artisans or low-paid factory workers (Karkhandar). They were not interested in education right from the beginning and the same trend continues even today.

MUSLIM WOMEN'S EDUCATION IN THE HISTORICAL PERSPECTIVE

As a result of this complex situation, the Muslim community remained in darkness in spite of so many changes in the recent years. Islam encourages learning. 'Iqra' (read) is the first word which worked as an instruction and was told to Prophet Mohammad (SAW) when the prophethood was conferred on him. Prophet Mohammad accorded the highest value to education. He said that "The ink of the Scholars is more holy than the blood of a Martyr" (Srivastava, 2003 : 5).

Ahmad rightly says in his detailed work on Muslim women, "Women proved their ability to master the literature... In the forefront was Al-khansa' the greatest poetess of her days, she was admired by the prophet himself" (Ahmad, 2003 : 89). Besides her, there were other outstanding women during those days, e.g.

- Zainab of Bani Awd tribe was a physician;
- Al-Shafa Bint Abdullah was appointed by the second caliph Hazrat Omar (R.A.A.) as superintendent of markets in Madina many times (Ahmad, 2003 : 89–90).

The status of women started deteriorating with the invasion of Mongols and Turks and ultimately the simple culture originated by Arab traditions was destroyed. Ahmad says, "the illiteracy of Muslim women reached its peak and became a widespread phenomenon in the world of Islam. Consequently women throughout the Muslim world became ignorant not only of outside affairs but also of their legal rights in terms of marriage, divorce and inheritance" (Ahmad, 2003: 93).

Muslims in India were equally or rather more deprived as compared with their counterparts from the other communities in the past. However, reformers made some efforts at the end of 19th century and a slow change was brought about among Hindus. Muslim reforms were initiated about eighty years later than Hindu reforms. They were started as efforts to curb social evils in Muslim society. Sir Syed Ahmad Khan the great educationist, tried to convince Muslims in favour of Western education. Beside his famous Muhammandan Anglo-Oriental College (which later took the shape of a university of world fame), he also established the Muhammandan Educational Conference which was started in 1886. It developed a separate wing for female education in 1906. This was initiated by one of the disciples of Sir Syed Ahmad Khan, Shaikh Abdullah who worked as secretary for the same organization. He started a monthly journal *'Khatoon'* in 1904 (Mohsini, 1987 : 90). The journal advocated female literacy. He along with his wife and sister-in-law established a school for girls where his wife and sister-in-law used to teach. The school was resisted by the orthodox lobby but later on got accepted. Begum Sultan Jahan donated liberally to the same. In 1925 it became an intermediate college and in 1937 a degree college. Now it is a famous women's college affiliated to Aligarh Muslim University. In fact, women's college deserves a special credit for Muslim women's education in north India. Thus Sir Syed's efforts were indirectly responsible for women's education and consequent improvement in their status. In other states also, Muslim women's education was encouraged during the same period. In the province of Punjab, Lady Girifth's Government High School and in Peshawar, Elizabeth High School were established for Muslim girls. Shekhawat Memorial Girls' School was founded at Calcutta (now Kolkata) in 1911. Maulvi Karamat Hussain established a girls' school at Lucknow in 1912 and Muslim ladies' Conference, Agra, started the Industrial

Training School for Muslim girls at the same time. One Urdu-medium school for girls was also established at Pune in 1913. The Nizam of Hyderabad Afzal-ul-Daula started several schools in the first and the second decade of the 20th century. Zanana College was established at Hyderabad in 1924.

Slowly and gradually, Muslim girls started understanding the importance of education. In Punjab *Anjuman-e-Himayat-I-Islam* started a degree college for women in 1939. In 1945 many Muslim girls submitted dissertations for M.A. and M.Ed. at the *Zanana College* (Srivastava, 2003 : 10).

Here, it is worth mentioning that Muslim women's education was particularly promoted by the British Government. It was reflected in 1854 Wood's Educational Despatch Concern. The grants-in-aid system was adopted during that time by the British government in India to promote and support schools started by Indians.

Governmental efforts are evident through the Hartong Committee which studied educational status of girls in British India in general and education of Muslim girls in particular. The Hartong Committee noted a significant increase in the enrolment of Muslim girls in schools during the decade 1917–27. It observed that in Punjab 17% of the school girls and 15% of the female college students were Muslims (Hartong Committee, 1929: 190–193). However, when we look at the whole of India, educated Muslim women were a micro scopic minority. Even then they had significant contribution and made their presence felt. Besides education and literacy, they were working on other fronts as well, for example, All India Muslim Ladies Conference which was initiated by the Begum of Bhopal at Aligarh in 1915, held its second session at Lahore in 1917. Here they passed a resolution against polygamy. Educated women themselves had been working for the education of Muslim girls. For example, Nawab Faizunnisa Chaudharani established an English-medium school for girls in 1873 in Bengal. It was meant for girls observing pardah. She set up primary schools in the whole of her estate. In 1882, 17000 girls were studying at the primary level, out of them 8.9% were Muslims. In 1931-32, the number of school-going girls was 5,35,000, out of them

56.6% were Muslims (Srivastava, 2003: 11).

In the beginning of the 20th century Madrasatul Banat was established at Delhi by famous Urdu fiction writer Allama Rashidul Khairi. It was a school-cum-hostel. Those days many Muslim girls who were getting education were also subscribing for women's periodicals such as *Tehzib-e-Niswan, Ismat,* etc. But this phase got over and the country was divided after some years. Partition and migration came as a big blow for the Indian Muslim communities. They felt displaced and rootless for sometime even without migrating, but soon, Muslims in independent India established themselves. However they remained conspicuously untouched by the winds of social change and social development.

It appears that lots of efforts have been made but in reality they could not make any visible dent in the educational scene of Indian Muslims. In 1981, the literacy rate among Muslims was 19%. The Eighth Annual Report (1985–86) of the Minorities Commission again mentions that Muslims are the most illiterate section. It has been found that in Muslim-managed schools also, non-Muslims keep on increasing and in the Board results they perform much better than Muslim students. The National Commission for Minorities' report for 1996–97 also reflects the same picture of Muslims' educational backwardness. It is to be noted that Muslims are not an insignificant minority. On 1 March, 2001, the Indian population crossed 1.02 crore, of which Muslims constitute around 12.52%. Many births in Muslim families remain unnoticed and un-registered. Therefore, some sections feel that Muslims in fact are nearly 18% of the Indian population. Increasing population among them means increasing incidence of illiteracy.

MUSLIM WOMEN'S EDUCATION AND THE NATIONAL SCENARIO

The size of an average Muslim household is larger than a non-Muslim household. Consequently, the Muslim population is growing faster. It was 9.91% in 1951, 10.69% in 1961, 11.21% in 1971, 11.35 in 1981, 12.12% in 1991and 12.52% in 2001. According to an NSS Report, average household size in rural areas for

Hindus is 4.9, for Muslims 5.6 and for Christians 4.4. For urban areas, average sizes of the households are 3.8, 4.4 and 5.5 for Christians, Hindus and Muslims respectively.

Notwithstanding the larger family size there are numerous socio-economic and political factors which account for educational backwardness of Muslims. Table 6.1 shows the literacy rate among Muslims.

Table 6.1

Per 1000 distribution of persons of age 15 years and above

All India

General education	*Religion*							
	1999–00				*1993–94*			
	Hinduism	*Islam*	*Christianity*	*all **	*Hinduism*	*Islam*	*Christianity*	*all**
	RURAL MALE							
not literate	368	409	241	369	410	473	224	411
literate & up to primary	255	303	307	260	274	303	336	276
middle	180	153	224	178	155	126	23	154
secondary	108	82	145	108	90	53	137	89
higher secondary	53	30	49	51	44	26	45	42
graduate & above	35	21	34	33	27	19	34	26
all	1000	1000	1000	1000	1000	1000	1000	1000
	RURAL FEMALE							
not literate	658	664	370	648	719	710	362	708
literate & up to primary	169	199	259	175	160	193	288	166
middle	96	89	165	98	70	68	176	73
secondary	48	32	123	50	34	20	116	36
higher secondary	19	10	49	19	12	5	40	12
graduate & above	9	4	33	9	5	2	18	5
all	1000	1000	1000	1000	1000	1000	1000	1000

				URBAN MALE				
not literate	129	259	60	146	145	292	56	162
literate & up to primary	187	274	140	198	225	298	216	233
middle	190	197	218	192	185	174	210	184
secondary	197	137	263	191	179	128	247	175
higher secondary	121	73	138	115	118	58	120	110
graduate & above	174	60	180	158	147	49	152	134
all	1000	1000	1000	1000	1000	1000	1000	1000
				URBAN FEMALE				
not literate	306	445	122	318	347	526	142	363
literate & up to primary	188	245	159	194	213	239	206	216
middle	160	140	200	158	146	113	195	143
secondary	145	90	222	141	130	73	238	127
higher secondary	90	45	146	86	77	30	105	72
graduate & above	109	34	150	101	85	19	112	78
all	1000	1000	1000	1000	1000	1000	1000	1000

Source: NSS Report No. 468, Employment and Unemployment Among Religion Groups in India 1999-2000.

It is surprising that numbers in the second category show a favourable trend for Muslims in all the four tables. In fact, this includes Quranic literacy which is compulsory for all Muslims. At least 95% Muslim childrens are sent to a teacher for learning Quranic recitation. It may be considered as initial literacy.

The table 6.1 shows that in the past years some improvement has taken place. Even then, the figures indicate that school attendance rate, in all age groups is the lowest among Muslims and highest among Christians. Nevertheless the difference between Muslims and non Muslims is constant in spite of some improvement in attendance rate in both the groups.

Abu Sualeh Sharif's Human Development Report (1999) gives some more statistics.

Table 6.2 : Rate of Literacy among children of 7 years and more

Religion	*Boys*	*Girls*
Hindu	65.90	39.20
Muslim	59.50	38.00
Christian	85.00	76.50
Other minorities	62.90	43.80

(quoted by Hamid, 2000)

Table 6.2 reflects the lowest achievement of Muslim children in the educational field. But in this age group the difference is not shocking.

At this juncture, one should look at the steps taken by the government. Education for everyone or equalization of educational opportunities is one of the primary concerns of the government. Many programmes have been launched for educationally backward communities during the past few decades. The foundation of our educational policy was laid down by the Articles 14, 29, 30, 340 and 350 of the Constitution. Some concrete steps have been taken up during last few years but even then Muslim women are not able to take the advantage of the positive trend and supportive measures.

FACTORS RESPONSIBLE FOR MUSLIM WOMEN'S EDUCATIONAL BACKWARDNESS

During the last decade of 20th century, the world changed tremendously. The situation in many Muslim countries improved in favour of women. But Indian Muslims are still marginalized deprived and backward. Education is their weakest point. General educational backwardness of Indian Muslims is more severely reflected in the case of women's education.

Let us examine the reasons for Muslim women's educational backwardness. Like all other social realities, educational backwardness of Indian Muslims is also an outcome of many complex factors. Some of these factors are as follows :-

- General poverty of Muslims compels them to discontinue their education at an early age and take up

- Voluntary action is the most important measure to improve the contemporary ethos. Efforts should begin with awareness generation and social education. Slowly and gradually vision of the whole community should be changed.
- Universalization of education with *Mahila Samakhya* and *Serv Shiksha Abhiyan* is very significant. It should be made mandatory for parents to send their children to school. Government bodies should develop a system to monitor regularity and attendance of all male and female children.
- Provision of quality education should be a priority for the government. Education should be made child friendly. It is important for all children but it is crucial for those who are even otherwise reluctant to attend school.
- Introduction of supervised home work classes and coaching centres should be one of the priority concern of NGOs. This helps in fulfilling the gaps in the learning process. It is particularly required for the first-generation learners.
- Vocational training courses and training-cum-production centres should be established and encouraged to make girls active in the field of learning and earning. Even otherwise, the relation between education and economic impendence must be highlighted.
- With the help of *Rashtriya Mahila Kosh*, special loans should be provided to the girls of backward communities for completing higher education and vocational training courses.
- For all the innovative educational projects at the time of campaign, religious leaders should be involved. Their statements and *Fatwas* carry great significance for illiterate and half literate people. If they project a positive picture, the masses get easily convinced, be it education or status of women.

CONCLUSION

It is pathetic that illiteracy has become a tradition for Muslim women. It is surprising that illiteracy is so common in this section in spite of the age-old practice of learning the Quranic script, which is not very different from Urdu. Quite a few of them learn recitation of the Holy Quran but many of them do not learn Urdu language. Other languages like Hindi or English are not even considered. Illiteracy, poverty, population explosion and shabby and sub-standard living make their lives miserable. This situation creates problems not only for them but also for the whole society. Besides the indifference of religious leaders, absence of political will is also responsible for this depressing state of affairs. Appeasement policy and lip service to the Muslim community is common at every level but proper and meaningful support is by and large missing. Muslims are used as a vote bank and after election they are ignored.

In the end, it is important to note that instead of blaming others, the Muslim community must start working on a self help basis. It is obvious that religious, political, social and economic forces are not supporting their development. They may be blamed for that but the exercise of putting blame or fixing responsibility on someone will not help the hopeless situation. Ultimately the sufferers will have to stand up and help themselves. Quality education and vocational/ professional training for women will definitely assist the whole community in getting proper share in the fruits of social development, as we know that only these get rewarded who strive for it.

REFERENCES

Ahmad, N. (2003). *Women in Islam* Vol. I, New Delhi, APH Publishing Corporation.

Hameed, S. S. (2000). Voice of the Voiceless, New Delhi, Report of the National Commission of Women.

Hartong Committee, (1929).

Indian Statutory, (Simon) Commission. (1929). *Report of the Educational Sub Committee*, Hartong Sub Committee 1929, London.

Mohsini, S.R. (1987). Social Reform Among Muslims, *Encyclopedia of Social Work*, Vol II, Government of India, Ministry of Welfare.

NSS Report. (2002). NSS 55th Round, Government of India Publication.

Srivastava, G. (2003). *The Legend Makers. Some Eminent Muslim Women of India*, New Delhi, Concept Publishing Company.

Chapter 7

The Status of Jain Women: Stated Ideals, Lived Realities

Manisha Sethi

This paper seeks to examine the continuities and ruptures between the stated ideals of womanhood in the large body of Jain literature and the reality of women's lives. My attempt will be to explore how dominant religious ideologies serve to disempower women in both the religious and secular domains, hoping to raise in the process, questions and issues that are central to the National Policy for Empowerment of Women.

Reports or scholarly works on the status of women within the Jain community are scarce, Jainism itself being till very recently a much-neglected domain of study.[1] Such a situation arises, I suspect, largely because Jains can appear to be largely indistinguishable from the surrounding caste Hindu society. This is slightly ironic because Jainism emerged as a challenge to the orthodox Brahminical practices and offered, at least theoretically, an alternative ideology of spiritual emancipation to groups—such as women and lower castes—which were hitherto outside the spiritual fold. Thus we will also investigate how far the general attitudes towards women remain similar or different from the wider caste Hindu attitudes. My attempt therefore will be to point to those areas of study which need further attention and hint at issues that must be addressed while formulating a policy for empowerment of women.

While spread in small numbers throughout the country, the Jains are mainly concentrated in three regions: The Deccan in the South; a wide band stretching across north-western India straddling the states of Gujarat and Rajasthan; and the areas of Punjab, Haryana and Madhya Pradesh. The last area encompasses Delhi, the eastern parts of Rajasthan and neighbouring parts of Madhya Pradesh. It should also be noted that the Jains are a predominantly urban community, more urban than any other group than perhaps the Zoroastrians. About 74.26 per cent of Jain population is concentrated in towns and cities with a mere 25.74 per cent residing in villages (The Census of India, 1991)[2]. The major economic activity that the Jains have traditionally engaged in is trading; this derives from the extreme emphasis laid in Jainism on the principle of *ahimsa* or non-violence, which rendered many vocations that involve some forms of violence as undesirable, even repugnant.

Further, Jains are not a homogenous whole but riddled with internal schisms. The most important division is the one between Svetambars and Digambars. The Svetambars, literally 'white clad', are the ones whose ascetics wear white clothes, while the Digambar monks are 'sky clad' and go naked. These are not mere matters of sartorial preference but have important theological underpinnings, as will soon become clear. The Svetambars are further subdivided into Murtipujaks (Tapaghaccha and Khartargaccha), Terapanthi and Sthanakvasis.

The presence of these cleavages, caste and sub-caste groups, and the Jain practice of intermarriages with Hindus has confounded anthropologists leading to much ink-spewing over whether Jains constitute a community or not in their own right, with defined boundaries and distinguishable features. In a pioneering collection of essays, the editors Michael Carrithers and Caroline Humphrey (1991) lay out a five-fold criteria which can justify the use of the term 'community' to define the Jains. These criteria are:

1. That the Jains themselves must share "in some significant sense, a common culture, belief, and practice, as well as some common interests".

2. Further, the Jains must be "significantly different from the surrounding society in their culture, beliefs, practices, and interests".
3. Recognising the inadequacy of the above two criteria, Carrithers and Humphrey emphasise the Jains' self consciousness "of an identity as Jains".
4. In keeping with the authors' requirement that a community be a distinct social entity and causal agent, the Jains "must be effective as a collectivity in social, political, and/or economic life".
5. Lastly, the authors demand that as a community, the Jains "must be able to reproduce itself".[3]

Needless to say, no localised community will be able to pass the Carrithers and Humphrey test. And therefore, not surprisingly, scholars who responded to the position paper forwarded by the duo appear at first instance to be contradicting each other. Christine M. Cottam Ellis, for instance, in her study of Jain merchants in a small town near Jaipur finds the category of Jains insufficient while J. Howard M. Jones finds it so in the study of Svetambar Jain merchants in a much smaller town in South Rajasthan (See Cort's "Recent Fieldwork Studies of the Contemporary Jains" in *Religious Studies Review*, Volume 23, Number 2, April 1997, p. 104.).

PART I

My focus on the debate over the status of Jains might seem to some as protracted and out of context here, but on closer examination it will be clear that women are central to any notion of community consciousness, and the nature of boundary formation of the Jain community has a direct bearing upon the status of Jain women. Beyond academic confines, the issue of whether Jains constitute an exclusive minority group or are a part of the larger Hindu majority has always been a contentious one and is most starkly foregrounded in the twin contexts of legal judgements and the census exercise.

Since the early days of the census, the British judges decreed that the Jains, like the Sikhs and Parsees, had "nothing or next to nothing in common with Brahminical worship" and that they could not be governed by Hindu law since "the term Hindu means persons within the purview of the *Shastras* which are at the bottom of Hindu law" (See *The Jains* by Paul Dundas, Routledge, 1992, London, pp. 4–5). The earliest censuses however, suggest that a large number of Jains preferred to regard themselves as Hindus. Sangave has noted an increasing communitarian consciousness by the beginning of the 20th century when Jains began to regard themselves as a distinct community (*Jain Community: A Social Survey* by V. A. Sangave, 1980, p. 3).

Legal pronouncements remained muddied, adding little to our understanding of the relationship between Jainism and Hinduism. While the Privy Council of 1921 declared that the Jains being Hindu dissenters would be judged by Hindu law, six years later the Chief Justice of the High Court dismissed such an assumption (Dundas, op. cit, 1992, London, p. 5). It is important to note, however, that the question of the legal standing of Jains as a distinct community was an essentially gendered question, at the heart of which lay the specifically Jain legal practice of widow inheritance in contra-distinction to the Hindu jurisprudence where the son or the close male agnates of the deceased inherit his property. This law was laid down in *Badrabahu Samhita*, a Digambar text but one which was accepted by the Svetambars as well. Not only did the deceased's widow inherit the dead man's property; she also enjoyed absolute and final authority over its use and disposal. Josephine Reynell has provided an account of the litigation that ensued (prior to the 1937 Hindu Woman's Right to Property Act), whereby the dead man's relatives petitioned the court to be governed by the Hindu law of succession and inheritance so as to gain control over the property in place of the widow. She cites instances where the court's ruling was in favour of the widow on grounds that Jains "are not governed by Hindu law in matters of adoption or the widows, right to adopt, as also in matters of succession and inheritance" ("Equality and Inequality" by Josephine Reynell in *Ideal, Ideology and Practice: Studies in Jainism*, edited by N.K. Singhi, 1987, p. 55).

It was seldom so simple though, and here we might benefit from examining some of the cases brought in the High Courts as recorded in *All India Reporters*. The litigation centres on the following issues:

1. Whether Jains would be governed by Hindu Law in matters of adoption. The courts recognised that the Jains completely disregard the *shraddha* ceremony and the sacrifice so essential in the instance of Hindus, thus rendering the matter of adoption a temporal or worldly rather than a religious issue. An important element of the cases I found was the issue whether a sonless widow could adopt without the direction or permission of her deceased husband.
2. Whether a Jain widow, in contrast to a Hindu widow, enjoyed greater rights as regards to inheritance of her dead husband's property. Here, a distinction was often made between self-acquired property of the husband and the ancestral property as is made in the case of the Hindu law.
3. Following from the above, the third important question or point of contest was whether the widows enjoyed the right to alienate the property so inherited in favour of either individuals (usually adopted sons) or religious and charitable trusts, i.e., if they could exercise an absolute interest in the estate.

In the *Sheokuabai v. Jeoraj* case, the Privy Council ruled that the "Jains so far have adopted the Hindu Law that the Hindu rules of adoption are applied to them in the absence of some contrary usage" (cited in Parshotam v. Venichand, *All India Reporter*, Bombay, 1921, 147, p. 148 and other cases) and this became the touchstone for all judgements that followed it. Deviations from Hindu Law were allowed in the case of Jains, provided an ancient and invariable custom was established with "the burden of establishing its antiquity and invariability ...on the parties averring its existence" (ibid. p. 150). Thus each case/suit became a sort of battleground to weld and prove the existence of a hoary tradition that offered better rights to

Jain women in general and Jain widows in particular or to disprove the existence of such a tradition. This resulted in a great diversity of judgements. In 1878, in the cases Sheo Singh Rai v. Dakho and Bhagvandas Tejmal v. Rajmal, the Privy Council ruled that the question whether "among the sect of the Jains known as Saraogi Agarwalas a sonless widow could adopt without permission from her husband or consent of his kinsmen and whether she could adopt the daughter's son was one which had been rightly held to be proved by the evidence given in the case" (ibid. 150). In the case of Prem Sagar v. Ram Gopal and others in 1929, the Court ruled that although a Jain widow, Mt. Gujri was not authorized to adopt a son in the absence of her husband's authority because the plaintiff could not demonstrate the proof of custom (Prem Sagar v. Ram Gopal and others, *All India Reporter*, Lahore, 814, pp. 814–815). In 1932 however, the Judge held that "there are on the present record the following 12 instances, proved by oral evidence of respectable witnesses, of valid adoptions by Jain widows of Delhi, the adoption in each case having been made long after the death of the husband and without authority from him or consent of kinsmen....A number of leading members of the Jain brotherhood have appeared as witnesses and deposed to the above custom, the most important of whom is R.S.P.D. Ram Chand, who is the Secretary of the local Jain Digambar Society."[4] The court concluded "beyond doubt that among Jains of Delhi, Hindu law has been varied to this extent that for adopting a son to her deceased husband, a widow need not possess express or implied authority from him, nor is the consent of the kinsmen necessary for the purpose." Note that it is 'respectable' members of the Jain 'brotherhood' who were recognized by the colonial courts as the legitimate representatives of their community with the powers to validate a customary practice. To this question of authentic voices of the community and its relationship to law, especially that which governs women and their rights, we shall return shortly.

Though dealing primarily with the issue of the legal right of the Jain widow to adopt, some of the cases throw light on the inheritance practices of the Jains and the legal view taken by the colonial courts. Gopi Mal and another v. Pannalal and others is one such case (*All India Reporter*, 1924, Lahore 339, pp. 339–342). The parties in the said dispute were Jains from Amritsar. Briefly the case was this: A house and half a share in a shop belonged to Kanshi Ram. He died leaving this to his wife who thereupon adopted a boy named Amin Chand and executed a will in his favour, appointing Amin Chand's natural father Gopi Chand as the manager. Following her death and till his own death, Amin Chand (the boy) remained in Gopi Chand's care after which Gopi Chand came in possession of the entire estate. The collaterals of deceased Kanshi Ram were demanding a share in the property while Gopi Chand was claiming an exclusive right over it as an inheritor of his dead son's property. If one were to read the case closely, it would reveal that the points of dispute were the following:

(*a*) whether an adoption among the Jains takes place in the *dattaka* form, where the adopted son becomes the full member of his adoptive family, or in the *Kritima* form, where the adopted son continues to retain ties with his natural family;

(*b*) whether Gopi Chand acted as a ward or trustee for his natural son.

What was beyond doubt and dispute was that Uttam Devi, the widow of Kanshi Ram inherited her dead husband's estate, and not his collaterals. She was the 'sole owner' who was entitled to execute a deed of adoption and a will in favour of her adopted son. The dead man's collaterals could stake a claim only upon the death of the widow and her adopted son.

One of the most interesting cases was Bhikubai Chunilal Ambaidas v. Manilal Bhagchand Raychand (*All India Reporter*, 1930, Bombay, 517, pp. 517–527). The suit not only mirrors the patriarchal anxiety about widow inheritance and their right to alienate such property but also highlights how the colonial state dealt with the relation between custom and law, how it mapped communities into neat slots, and how it came to recognize and evolve a criteria for establishing the validity of custom and practice in order to frame laws and arbiter justice to the native population. The outlines of the suit are as follows: Rupchand died in 1906 leaving behind him two sonless widows and mother Chunabai. According to the will executed by Rupchand, his mother was appointed manager of his property; his wives were to act according to her directions. Chunabai, following the death of the two widows, succeeded to the estate and executed a deed of will in favour of her daughter's daughter, Bhikubai, the defendant in the suit. The defendant's case was that "the parties were Jains [Dasha Shrimali Shvetambar Jains], and according to the Jain law and custom of the caste Rupchand's widows became the heirs and absolute owners of Rupchand's property, and after the death of the widows, Chunabai, the mother of Rupchand, according to the Jain law and the custom of the caste, became the absolute owner, and further that by his will dated..., Rupchand had constituted Chunabai as the absolute owner and the defendant obtained title to the property under the gift deed of Chunabai..."(ibid. p. 518).

An appeal is made to the "Jain law and custom of the caste" in order that the parties in suit be treated differently from the Hindu law. More specifically that Jain widows unlike Hindu widows have absolute rather than partial interest in the estate of their dead husband/son. Thus in the Judge's view, "the only question in this case is whether the custom set up by the defendant that Rupabai and Motibai, the widows of Rupchand, took an absolute estate and Chunabai, the mother, also took an absolute estate and was competent to pass the deed of gift and the will... is proved" (ibid. p. 519). In order to authenticate the custom, the Judge laid out for examination four kinds of evidence: earlier judicial evidence, ancient Jain texts, opinion evidence and instance evidence. Twenty-seven court decisions from different High Courts and of the Privy Council were drawn upon. Without going into the details of each case discussed—which were sometimes conflicting—suffice it to say that the Judges came to the conclusion that it could not be held that the Jain widow either enjoyed an absolute estate or the right to alienate immovable property which was part of the ancestral estate though some earlier judgements had conceded the right of the widow over her dead husband's self acquired property.

The Judges rejected a reliance upon ancient Jain texts, such as the Badrabahu Samhita, Arhan Niti and Vardhaman Niti, all of which recognize the widow as an heir to her dead husband's property on grounds of inconsistency and mutual contradiction[5]. More importantly, they held that the rules of inheritance and succession laid out in these texts are obsolete and "relate to a condition of Jain society when the widow was considered as a more preferential heir than the son, and cannot have any binding force at the present time" (ibid. p. 519).

Thus, the Jain widows had "no better rights than a widow" (ibid. p. 524) and would be ruled by the Mitakshara law. Although the Judge began by placing no great importance on the vexed question of the status of Jains as a community, towards the end of the judgement, it was clearly spelled out that Jains being Hindu dissenters should be governed by Hindu Laws (ibid. p. 521).

This was further ossified when, following Independence, the constitution makers in Article 25 stated that "when the term 'Hindu' and 'Hinduism' are used within the Constitution, they are to be taken to include the Jains" (Dundas, op.cit., p. 4). Likewise the Hindu Law Committee brought the Jains under the purview of the Hindu Personal Law, rejecting the validity of a separate legal code. Recently, some states have granted Jains the status of a minority, it is to be seen what impact this might have on the debate on personal laws.

PART II

One of the most striking features of Jainism is that it opened for women the possibility of joining its ascetic orders; women comprise a vital component of the fourfold Jain schema called the *caturvidhasangha* which divides the society into *sadhus, sadhvis, shravaks* and *shravikas* (laymen and women). In South Asian religions the most appropriate and codified religious roles proffered to women lie within the domain of the household, the primary moral and religious duty of a married woman being *pativratadharma*. Jainism provided an institutional mechanism for women to pursue their spiritual goals autonomously outside the context of kin and family roles.

Even more startling is the visible preponderance of the women ascetics over the male ascetics. From Table 7.1, it is self evident that the statistics are heavily skewed in favour of female ascetics, except in the case of Digambars (Figures of 1998 from Jain samgra Chaturmas Suchi cited in "Women and Jainism in India" by Nalini Balbir in *Women in Indian Religions* edited by Arvind Sharma).

TABLE 7.1 : Male and Female Asceties among Jains

	Monks	*Nuns*	*Total*
Svetambars Murtipujaks	1474	5420	6894
Sthanakvasis	536	2638	3174
Terapanthis	147	538	685
Digambars	415	350	765

Sources such as the *Kalpasutra* are clear that on Mahavira's death, the *tirtha* that he had founded contained a body of female ascetics two and a half times as large as the number of male ascetics and a lay community containing twice as many laywomen as laymen. Not only this, the number of women who are described as achieving *moksha* also outstrips the number of men. Further, it is also a woman, Marudevi, who bears the distinction of being the first person in this world age to have attained liberation.

Spiritually heroic women comprise an oft-repeated theme in Jain literature and there exists a veritable body of commentaries and secondary sources that have described in detail the complementary references to women. *Jina matas*, or mothers of the Jinas (the venerable ford makers) are the most revered. Women who overcame opposition to practise their faith are the staple heroines of sagas penned by the ascetics[6].

In this section, we will briefly survey the Jain literature to interrogate the position of women within it. The Jain literature dealing with the question of woman's capacity or incapacity for spiritual liberation is a useful source for examining traditional attitudes towards women and sexuality. This shall be juxtaposed with assertions of some Jain nuns to give an idea of the prevailing notions. Towards the end, I will draw upon my own fieldwork experience among Jain nuns in Delhi, Agra and Jaipur, hailing from various Jain sects.[7] In conjunction they reveal the patriarchal biases of religions, even those that espouse the spiritual equality of genders. I emphasise the voices of the Jain *sadhvis* because unlike the *sadhvis* in Hindu society, they are not marginal figures but central to the perpetuation of the community's religious and social life; they play an important part in what Carrithers and Humphrey identify as an important criteria for justifying Jains as a community, namely, the "reproduction of Jainism".[8] Again the discordant voices of the *sadhvis* underscore the important point that religion is not merely a set of abstract ideas but lived reality and with changing times, both religion and patriarchy may be reformulated.

The figure of the religious woman—the ascetic as well as the lay—has been used to define the boundaries and self-identity of the community. The question of women and salvation has formed the core of polemics between the Digambars and the Svetambars as "a kind of protracted metaphor for a struggle over the spiritual validity of the two paths of Jain mendicancy" (Dundas, op. cit., p. 48). The Digambars insisted that ascetic prerequisite to the path of liberation and the woman's inability to shed clothes excluded them from ascetic lives and consequently enlightenment. Their continued attachment to clothes indicated that they could never be free from the powerful emotions of shame and fear arising from their naked bodies. While accepting the impossibility of female nudity, *Shaktayana*, a Svetambar text dismisses the centrality of nudity in the development of religious life. Indeed the Svetambars depict the 19th *Tirthankara* or ford maker, Malli, as a woman.

The crux of the arguments forwarded by Digambars against the possibility of women to achieve liberation, while numerous and multi-pronged, hinge on the peculiar female physiology. The most commonly cited reasons are women's physical, moral, intellectual and ethical inferiority. Women have fewer bones than men and are therefore unsuited to extreme austerities regarded as indispensable for liberation; in the crevices of her body parts, especially genitals, space between her breasts and arm pits nestle millions of tiny microbes called *apryaptas*, which the woman by her sheer ordinary, day-to-day activities destroys. The sin of such large-scale, albeit involuntary, violence must be borne by the woman. The very femaleness of the woman is a source of the greatest violation of Jain principal of non-violence. There arises here a contradiction between the high spiritual status accorded to women on par with men and the strong gynophobia that underlies many of the pronouncements and assumptions in the Jain literature. As in Brahminical texts, women are often cast as evil temptresses that mislead the male spiritual aspirants from the path of salvation. Several texts issue warnings to monks about the inherently wicked nature of women:

> "...with crafty, stealthy step, sweet-spoken women; they know how to contrive that some monks will suffer a (moral) breakdown. They sit down closely at his side, they frequently put on holiday dress, they show him even the lower part of their body and the armpit when lifting their arm...He should not fix his eyes on those (women), nor should he consent to (women's) inconsiderate acts, nor should he walk together with them: thus his soul is well-guarded."

(cited in "Women in Jainism" by Nalini Balbir in *Women and Religion* edited by Arvind Sharma, 1987, p. 130).

Whilst there is a complete absence of similar passages warning women/nuns of the dangers of male sexuality, J.C. Jain gives a solitary reference that implicates both men and women equally for infirmity of moral strength.

> "The faults that are indicated in women are also noticed in men, perhaps in a larger quantity in men who are more powerful. As men are condemned by virtuous women so are women by virtuous men. Both gain eminence on account of their virtues... As a matter of fact, one gets deteriorated by one's own laxity whether man or woman."

(Acharya Sivakoti in *Bhagavati Aradhna*, quoted in "The Status of Women in Jain Literature" by J.C. Jain in *Ideal, Ideology and Practice: Studies in Jainism* edited by N.K. Singhi, 1987, p. 144–45).

Such references are however an exception than a rule.

Several nuns I spoke to echoed the view that women are by nature fickle-minded and bearers of an unbridled sexuality that inevitably led to the spiritual downfall of men. While narrating the tale of Muni Sthulbhadra, Sadhvi Prafullprabha emphasised as much to me. In her own words:

> "...Sthulbhadra Muni lived with a prostitute for twelve years. But later, he changed and thought that he should convert the prostitute into a pious shravika. When he returned [with this aim], the prostitute thought that he had come back to her. Upon seeing him she exclaimed that he, who used to appear like a prince earlier with his fine clothes and jewellery, was looking like a beggar. The Muni replied that he had renounced the world and become an ascetic. The prostitute mocked at him and challenged him to observe his chaturmas in her pleasure palace. So the muni spent his chaumasa in that pleasure palace which had erotic pictures painted on its walls. The prostitute danced before him and brought him rich food—but he remained stoic/ unmoved. His was only one aim—that of converting the prostitute to shravika, to bring her to the true path and finally he succeeded.
>
> Sthulbhadra's guru had four disciples: one spent his chaturmas near a lion's den; another near a snake's pit, the third on the periphery of a deep well. But upon hearing them all, the guru declared that Sthulbhadra's had been the most severe because he had won over a woman. If one sees, all of these were very dangerous but Sthulbhadra's was by far the most dangerous. Even great Munis can fall from their greatness [because of women]."[9]

Women's bodies are seen as constituting the locus of violence and sexual desire—the very antithesis of Jainism. Despite its associations with fecundity, menstrual blood has terrifying qualities in mythology and religious literature[10]. According to the Digambar view recorded in a 17th-century text,

> "Women, namely those beings who have the physical sign of

> the human female, do not attain moksha in that very life for their souls do not manifest that pure transformation which is called a "perfect being"… biologically the female is distinguished … by the fact that she has an impure body, as is evident by the flow of menstrual blood each month."

This view is neither archaic nor restricted to the Digambars, it was espoused by the more liberal Svetambars as well. It should be noted too that the most stringent critique of the Digambar position was provided not by the Svetambars but by a small sect, now extinct, called the Yapaniya. Indeed Sadhvis of the Tapagach told me of the rigorous taboos they observed during the days of the menstrual cycle: they do not participate in any religious activity; sit aloof from others; do not go out for their daily round of *gochri* or alms collection; do not touch anything, especially religious texts as knowledge is said to take leave during this period. This might be one of the reasons why *sadhvis* of the Tapagach are the least educated. Sadhvi Dinmani attributed particularly morbid features to the menstrual cycle.

> "...we consider it absolutely impure. During this time we do not read any Sutras. We even recommend complete silence. If you utter any words during the menstrual cycle you accrue sins. …if you are in the samsara, then you should not cook or enter the kitchen, it kills all the food. Nurses are not allowed to enter the operation theatre if they are bleeding, the operation may go wrong. Even savouries may be destroyed if prepared by women having menses. The papads may turn red. … Flowers may wilt if tended to by women having menses..."

Notwithstanding the fact that both monks and nuns are subject to the same discipline regime and there are no distinctions in terms of training and learning, there is a clearly established hierarchy. The relations between the nuns and monks seem to mimic the gendered relations of super-ordination and subordination in a domestic setting. The nuns are expected to show deference to the monks and even the most senior nun must remain submissive to even the most junior monk's authority. The *prabartini* who heads the order of the nuns is subject to the authority of the *acharya* who heads the order of the monks. Moreover, a nun is precluded from the possibility of attaining the status of an *acharya*. The nuns are prohibited from undertaking the study of *Mahaparijna, Arunopapata* and the *Drstivada,* being of "fickle mind" (Sangave, op. cit., p. 170).

Even Mallinath, the only female ford maker is invariably represented in androgynous terms with the diacritical marks of her sex conspicuously absent. Indeed the story of Mallinath goes that Malli was in a previous birth a prince called Mahabal and was reborn as a woman as punishment for a sin in that past birth!

One *sadhvi* of the Khartargach, when questioned about the unequal nature of such an arrangement replied that though the soul has no gender, these institutional mechanisms are necessary to regulate society, and the monastic orders were part of the social world. While many *sadhvis* hailing from Digambar path and Tapagacha, Khartartgach and Terpanthi upheld such a discriminatory hierarchical order, there is a group of nuns from the reformist Sthankavasis which has resisted and reinterpreted the teachings of the Jinas to argue for a more egalitarian institutional structure. At the focus of their ire has been the practice of *vandana* or paying obeisance to male mendicants regardless of their age. At a *sammelan* of the Sthanakvasis held at Pune in 1987, *Sadhvi* Dr. Manjushri ji led a minor movement against the practice.[11] She called a separate meeting attended by seventy-seven *sadhvis* prior to the main council in which a resolution against *vandana vyavhar* was passed. But, according to Dr. Manjushri, the nuns were reprimanded by their male gurus and withdrew support to this resolution soon after. She and her disciples no longer bow to sadhus younger to them. According to her, the appeal to scriptural authority is misplaced, as there is no Shastric validation for this practice; it is the male quest for domination that lies at the heart of this:

> "One *sadhu* said to me, today you are demanding that this rule should be scrapped, tomorrow you shall demand that *sadhvis* be made *Acharya*. I replied that certainly we shall demand that too—it is our right. He said that is precisely why we do not concede your demand [on *vandana vyavhar*].

> They [the *sadhus*] are afraid; they fear the loss of power because we are numerically stronger. So they wish to perpetuate this order.

Once while I was discussing these issues with a group of *sadhvis* at a *sthanak* in Gurgaon, a young *sadhvi* turned to her Guruni and asked why, if in Mahavir's time Chandanbala could lead thousands of *sadhvis*, there were no women *acharyas* in present times.[12] Some groups have indeed broken this taboo and made *sadhvis acharya*—*Acharya* Sadhna of the Arhat Sangh in Delhi and *Acharya* Chandana in Rajgir are examples of this.

As noted earlier, nuns act as moral guides for the community, especially for the lay women who spend at least some part of their day at the *upasray*/temple or *sthanak* where a group of *sadhvis* might be staying. The story of Sthulbhadra or Rajul and her brother-in-law[13] therefore are not mere tales but laid out as ideals of womanhood for the *shravikas* to follow. *Sadhvi* Prafullprabha ended her tale by reiterating that women are the cause of moral degradation of today's men. "Look at the boys of today. They have all been spoilt by these girls...the way they dress, their bodies, their behaviour...what do the boys have? Women are the cause of spoiling men." The story of Maina Sundari who by the heat of her austerities was not only able to miraculously cure her leper husband but also convert her unbelieving father into a devout *shravak* was narrated to me in the context of explaining to me the correct wifely and religious roles of a woman. *Sadhvi* Sayam ratna Shri ji concluded this by drawing a comparison of the dutiful wife Maina Sundari who waited for her husband for several years (in which time the man had married 13 different women) with a Jain woman in the neighbourhood—a widow with two children—who had recently re-married.[14]

PART III

This brings us to the final part of this paper that attempts at understanding the status of Jain women in contemporary times through an analysis of certain social indicators and the prevailing socio-cultural norms regarding womanhood among the Jains.

Social Indicators

The sex distribution of Jain population clearly indicates a deficiency of women. According to the 1991 Census, there are only 946 women for every 1000 males, slightly higher than the 1971 figure of 940 females per 1000 male. This compares favourably with the all-India average of 927 females for every 1000 males.* Wastage of females is considerably less among the Jains in comparison with other communities. If one were to compare the Census figures of the number of male and female children born and the number of male and female children surviving, one could conclude that the chances of survival of a girl child are comparable to that of a male child. Sangave concurs that the discrepancy in the male–female ratio may be due to the fact that traditionally, Jain women marry early and are called upon to bear many children, resulting in higher female mortality in the age group of 5–40—also the age group which shows a lower number of females than males (Sangave, op. cit., p. 20).

Recent data suggests that for almost 25 per cent of Jain women in the urban areas and around 43 per cent in the rural areas, the average age of marriage continues to be below 17 years. Twenty per cent of the girls in the rural Jain population are married between the ages of 14 and 15.

The literacy rate for Jain women stands at a remarkable high of almost 79.36 per cent in urban areas and 61.9 per cent in rural areas.

Given below is the percentage distribution of literacy rates for Jain women at different levels:

Urban

Literate but below middle: 27.52%
Middle but below matric: 15.10%
Matric but below graduate: 24.94%
Graduate and above: 11.80%

---

* The 2001 Census shows that at an All India level the Sex ratio in 0–6 age group is 870, and in major states with large Jain population, the 0–6 sex ratio is low for instance 832 in Gujarat and 878 in Rajasthan.

Rural

Literate but below middle: 34.80%
Middle but below matric: 14.37%
Matric but below graduate: 11%
Graduate and above: 1.71%

Thus, a large proportion of these women who have studied have access to education only up to the matric level.

While the statistics on the whole do not look so bleak, indeed the Jain women appear to fare better than many other groups. Bald statistics by themselves do not always reflect the whole truth. These statistics should be seen in conjunction with the widespread ideals of womanhood in the society.

Several field studies have indicated that there exists a marked son preference among the Jains and women often visit temples in the hope of being granted this wish. Let us bear in mind here that there is no religious requirement for a male progeny in Jainism as in Hinduism where the *pindadana* offering by the son is essential for spiritual liberation. The gendered division of the religious duties however, reflects the power relations between the sexes. A man acquires spiritual merits through his acts of donations—either to the temples and other religious or social institutions—usually much publicised and ostentatious affairs in the community[15]; a woman gains merit by fasting. It points to the fact that control over the economic resources is exercised by men who alone can indulge in these acts of *dana* on behalf of their families. The dominant ideal for woman continues to remain that of a homebound subservient wife as Josephine Reynell's fieldwork among the Shvetambars also suggests. Women are not regarded as autonomous agents; even the right of the women to inherit and alienate the immoveable property was considered most legitimate and appropriate when done in favour of the religious institutions than for personal gains. The intensity of the campaign against widow inheritance provides proof that even ideals of female equality do not necessarily guarantee social equality for women.

CONCLUSION

In absence of empirical studies and other statistical evidence, it is difficult to give a conclusive account of the status of Jain women. My attempt in this paper was less ambitious—I sought to understand social and religious ideals about womanhood in Jainism and how they are played out in the context of everyday lives of the women. It was evident that even though a religion may be premised on the equality of the sexes, a monolithic model of such equality is hard to decipher. While Jainism opened its doors for women to pursue their spiritual goals, i.e., it offered spiritual equality, this did not translate into their social empowerment. Indeed even this spiritual equality became a battleground for sectarian hegemony with contesting claims about women's ability to achieve liberation. Indeed this running battle spawned some of the most misogynist religious literature in South Asia.

If anything, my paper points to the glaring paucity of research in the area and underlines the urgency of taking on the same.

NOTES

1. John E. Cort has noted with satisfaction the increasingly fecund field of Jain Studies with publication of a number of field work based studies on contemporary Jains (see "Recent Fieldwork Studies of the Contemporary Jains" in *Religious Studies Review*, Volume 23, Number 2, April 1997, pp. 103–111). These broadly focus on Jain social organisation and Jain ritual. There have also been some welcome historical and literary studies. See among others *The Assembly of Listeners: Jains in Society* edited by Michael Carrithers and Caroline Humphrey, 1991; *Riches and Renunciation: Religion, Economy, and Society among the Jains* by James Laidlaw, 1995; The *Archetypal Actions of Ritual: A Theory of Ritual Illustrated by the Jain Rite of Worship*, by Caroline Humphrey and James Laidlaw 1994; *Absent Lord: Ascetics and Kings in a Jain Ritual Culture* by Lawrence A. Babb, 1996 and *Open Boundaries: Communities and Cultures in Indian History* by John E. Cort, 1998, himself. For gender and Jainism, P.S. Jaini's masterly compilation of Jain debates on the subject, *Gender and Salvation: Jain Debates on the Spiritual Liberation of Women*,

1991 is indispensable. N. Shanta's magisterial *The Voice of the Unknown Sadhvi: The History, Spirituality and the Life of the Jaina Women Ascetics* surveys the social organisation and spiritual worldview of the Jain nuns. Kelting focuses on the religiosity of the lay women through a study of the women's bhajan mandals.

2. All data henceforth is derived from The Census of India, 1991 unless otherwise mentioned.
3. "Jains as a Community: A Position paper" by Michael Carrithers and Caroline Humphrey in *The Assembly of Listeners: Jains in Society* edited by Michael Carrithers and Caroline Humphrey (Cambridge University Press, Cambridge, 1991).
4. This suggests that the practice of sonless widows adopting sons without the permission of their husbands and kinsmen was common to both Digambars and Shvetambars.
5. Josephine Reynell suspects that the enshrinement of woman's right to inherit may not have derived from a commitment towards gender equality but from religious institutions instinct from self-preservation and perpetuation. She says that it was likely that many childless widows donated their inheritance to religion as an act of dana or charity. This contention is also supported by the litigation I delved into-often the widows alienated their inheritance in favour of religious institutions and charitable trusts. See Josephine Reynell, "Equality and Inequality" in N.K. Singhi (ed.) Ideal, Ideology and Practice: Studies in Jainism (Jaipur, Printwell Pub., 1987) pp. 55.
6. Nuns are prolific writers and their repertoire includes religious essays, polemical pieces, poetry and fiction. These books are often borrowed by lay women to read.
7. The fieldwork was conducted for my Ph.D Thesis on Jain nuns. I have tried to explore the possible reasons for the numerical preponderance of nuns among the Jains and interrogate the ideas of sexuality and renunciation.
8. I am not suggesting that the religion of the Jains is an unchanging historical stream and mendicants the only agents of change, but only that the mendicants and especially female mendicants, by the sheer power of their numbers and visibility, and their interactions with the laity are important in the community as disbursers of morality.
9. In personal conversation with Sadhvi Prafullprabha. She belongs to Tapagach and was initiated at the age of 13 years (on 22 February 1973). She has no formal education but is self-

taught and can read and write in Gujarati, Hindi and English.

10. See *Julia Leslie, "Menstruation Myths" in Leslie (ed.) Myths and Mythmaking* (Surrey, Curzon Press, 1996).
11. Dr. Manjushri in personal conservation. In recognition of her progressive outlook, she has been christened Jain Kranti (revolution).
12. Sadhvi Subhasha ji in personal discussion at the Jain School near Shvetambar Jain Sthanak, Gurgaon.
13. Rajul, the wife of Bhagwan Neminath was passing through a dense forest when it began to rain. She took refuge in a cave, not knowing her brother-in-law was meditating there. She took off her clothes to dry and this aroused the meditating man. When he approached her, Rajul prevailed upon him to turn back as she had been renounced by his brother, i.e., her husband. She was therefore akin to vomit. This story was narrated to me by Sadhvi Prafullprabha.
14. Sadhvi Sayam Ratna Shri ji was a widow herself when she took *diksha*. She belonged to the Tapagach. I have not verified the stories or characters with texts as I am interested not in the authenticity but the moral content of the narratives.
15. See James Laidlaw's *Riches and Renunciation: Religion, Economy and Society among the Jains* for the apparent contradiction between the high value attached to extreme asceticism in Jainism on the one hand, and the visible display of wealth, even, and especially in a religious context such as donation on the other.

REFERENCES

All India Reporter. (1921). Parshotam Ganpat Gujar-Plaintiff-Appellant v. Venichand Gujar-Defendant-Respondent, Bombay, 147.

All India Reporter. (1924). Gopi Mal and another-Appellants v. Pannalal and others-Respondents, Lahore, 339.

All India Reporter. (1929). Prem Sagar-Plaintiff-Appellant v. Ram Gopal and others-Defendants-Respondents, Lahore, 814.

All India Reporter. (1930). Bhikubai Chunilal Ambaidas-Defendant-Appellant v. Manilal Bhagchand Raychand-Plaintiff-Respondent, Bombay, 517.

All India Reporter. (1932). Mt. Lado-Plaintiff-Appellant v. Banarsi Das and others-Defendents-Respondents, Lahore, 546.

All India Reporter. (1932). Sundar lal-Plaintiff-Appellant v. Baldeo

Singh and others-Defendents-Respondents, Lahore, 426.

Balbir, N. (1987). "Women in Jainsim", in Arvind Sharma (ed.) Women and Religion, Albany: SUNY, 121–138.

Balbir, N. (2002). Indian Reprint, Arvind Sharma (ed.) Women and Religion, New Delhi: Oxford University Press, 70–107.

Carrithers, M. and Caroline H. (1991). "Jains as a Community: A Position paper" in Carrithers and Humphrey (eds.) *The Assembly of Listeners: Jains in Society*, Cambridge: Cambridge University Press.

Cort, J.E. (ed.) (1998). *Open Boundaries: Jain Communities and Cultures in Indian History*, New York: SUNY.

______1997. "Recent Fieldwork Studies of the Contemporary Jains" in *Religious Studies Review*, Volume 23, Number 2, April, 103–111.

Dundas, P. (1992). *The Jains*, London and New York: Routledge.

Jain, J.C. (1987). "The Status of Women in Jain Literature: An Analysis," in N.K. Singhi (ed.) *Ideal, Ideology and Practice: Studies in Jainism*, Jaipur: Printwell Publishers, 142–48.

Jaini, P.S. (1991). *Gender and Salvation: Jain Debates on the Spiritual Liberation of Women*, California: University of California Press.

Laidlaw, J. (1995). *Riches and Renunciation: Religion, Economy and Society among the Jains*, Oxford: Clarendon Press.

Leslie, J. (1996). "Menstruation Myths" in Leslie (ed.) *Myths and Mythmaking*, Surrey: Curzon Press.

Reynell, J. (1987). "Equality and Inequality", in N.K. Singhi (ed.) *Ideal, Ideology and Practice: Studies in Jainism*, Jaipur: Printwell Publishers, 33–58.

______(1991). "Women and Reproduction of the Jain Community," in Michael Carrithers and Caroline Humphry (eds.) *The Assembly of Listeners: The Jains in Society*, Cambridge: Cambridge University Press, 41–65.

Sangave, V.A. (1980). *Jain Community: A Social Survey.*

Chapter 8

Retired Women : Role Transition

Sushma Batra

'Social role' refers to the functioning of individuals in the group or the larger society. As an individual interacts with different groups, he learns his social roles. These vary with culture: individual's capacities, ability to adapt and situations. Roles played by individuals are highly significant. Ralph Linton (1968) defines social role as the sum total of the cultural patterns associated with a particular status including "the attitudes, values and behaviour ascribed by the society to any and all persons occupying this status". Thus, a status is a recognized and regulated position in a society. It offers some rules for what, how and with whom the person claiming that status is supposed to act. According to Linton, role involves the performance of the rights and duties constituting a particular status. He finds seven age-sex groupings in practically all societies: infant, boy, girl, adult man, adult woman, old man and old woman.

Heiss (1981) defines roles as the behavioural expectations of what a person "should" do. This "should" come from the expectations associated with established and recognized roles, with roles in informal and emergent situations, and with the person's own self-concept and inclinations.

Thus social roles could be described as patterns of behaviour that individuals are expected to display under certain conditions involving other people. In everyday life, all of us routinely occupy many statuses, both formal and informal, and enact complex repertoires of roles (Merton, 1957; Heiss, 1981). The sum of an individual's perceptions and evaluation of his roles constitutes his concept of "self". The person performing a role is called "role occupant" or a "role carrier".

The roles a person assumes and plays depend upon various factors such as age, mental status, physical condition, socio-economic and cultural background. These roles are different for different life phases. The individuals enter these roles with varying expectations. The ability to adapt to these roles depends upon their personality and their eagerness to perform the various role-related activities under that role. The more wholly they are involved, the more the "self" and the "role carrier" merge and become one. These roles are called vital/ primary roles and they gradually get internalized. A person learns through the primary group what the expectations for a given social role in the society are and the network of role relationships that this primary group provides normally prepares and tries to fulfil the role expectations. This process is called **role adaptation.**

CHANGE IN ROLES

These roles change over a period of time. According to Rosow (1976) the role change involves five different temporal connotations:

1. Shifting of Roles: The first is that of the simple movement between two positions that a person holds simultaneously, namely, moving between family and work role (role shift). These role changes involve routine shifts between different role relationships in a short time.

2. Modification of Roles: Roles may be modified and redefined as a function of social change. They are transformed in their content, normative expectations and so on in response to historical events. They usually occur over a period of time. For example, change in the role of parents in a joint family to their role in a nuclear family.

3. Change in Roles as Correlates of Age: These are comparable changes within single roles through time as correlates of age that are functions of different life stages, e.g. role changes as people traverse the life-cycle from childhood through adolescence, middle age, adulthood to old age.

4. Acquisition of New Roles and Losing Existing Ones: The alteration of the status set by the acquisition of new roles or relinquishment of the existing ones, e.g. an individual adds or loses a role by joining or leaving a group or association, whether formal or informal. This type of change is again age-related, as, depending on one's age the person may join a youth club and later shift to "senior citizen" club.

5. Role Change as Status Changes : This is related to one's status. For instance, the occupational status of a person comes to an end with mandatory retirement and the individual is forced to accept the new role of a "retiree". This role change is again related to one's age.

ROLE CHANGES THROUGH THE LIFE SPAN

The entire life-cycle can be viewed as a succession of roles (Seugarten and Datan, 1973). We are constantly acquiring, modifying and changing roles. The roles are age graded, i.e. at each stage certain characteristics must be acquired if the individual has to be successfully accepted as a member of society. Brim and Wheeler (1966) have described the socialization process throughout the life span. They stress the fact that different demands are placed on an individual by the environment/society and other individuals at different points of the life-cycle. Thus, the major factor that contributes to socialization involves the individual learning to anticipate the other individual's response to one's own behaviour, then reflecting upon this behaviour and judging it as either good or bad.

Erikson (1963), Havighurst (1972) and Hurlock (1980) subdivided the life span into various stages. Erikson named them as progressive stages, and divided them into eight stages. Havighurst called them development tasks (six tasks) and Hurlock used the term "periods" or stages (10 stages). Table 8.1 depicts the various stages/development tasks used by all the three researchers.

TABLE 8.1
Division of life span into various Stages/Periods

Erikson	*Havighurst*	*Hurlock*
Infancy (0–1) (Basic trust vs mistrust)	Babyhood and early childhood	Prenatal period : conception to birth
Early childhood (1–3 yrs) (Autonomy vs shame and doubt)	Late childhood	Infancy: birth to the end of the second week
Play age (3–6 yrs) (Initiative vs Guilt)	Adolescence	Babyhood: end of the second week to end of the second year
School age (6–12) (Industry vs inferiority)	Early adulthood	Early childhood: (2–6)
Adolescence (12–19) (Ego Identity vs Role confusion)	Middle adulthood	Late childhood: (6–12)
Early Adulthood (20–25) Intimacy vs Isolation	Middle age	Puberty or preadolescence: (10–14)
Adulthood (26–64) (Generativity vs Stagnation)	Old age	Adolescence: (13–18) teen or fourteen to
Later Adulthood (65–death) Ego Integrity vs Despair)		Early adulthood: (18–40)
		Middle Age (40–60 yrs) Old Age (60 to death)

Erikson contends that each stage has two possible resolutions, positive and negative. In all the stages, the negative crisis/conflict must be resolved if psychological development is to proceed normally. Similarly, Havighurst argued that the successful achievement of developmental tasks at a particular age, that leads to happiness and failure would lead to unhappiness and difficulty with later tasks. According to all, the scholars some tasks arise mainly in respect of physical maturation, others develop primarily from the cultural pressures of society and still others grow out of the personal values and aspirations of the individual.

All the individuals do not reach these stages at the same time and accomplish what they "should" at a particular age. Brim (1966) describes the process of adult socialization as distinctly different from that of childhood. Further, the contents and goals of the socialization process and behaviour are also different during adulthood.

During childhood, socialization agents tend to have an emotional and/or personal tie to the individual such as a parent, brother, sister, etc. During adulthood, however, socialization agents are mostly impersonal. They vary from being one's boss or any employer or third person acting as a role model for him. Therefore, during childhood these socialization agents are concerned with the child acquiring rules or values regulating behaviour. Its examples are non-stealing, working hard and being responsible. On the other hand, during adulthood, socialization agents are concerned with the adult acquiring specific role behaviours. Even the instruments designed to measure adjustments of younger individuals cannot be used to measure adjustments of older people.

With age, the status and role of an individual shifts. But with the onset of old age, many of these roles undergo a major change, some even disappear, e.g. the completion of child-rearing function, loss of spouse, loss of work and change in familial status and role. These roles can neither be replaced nor compensated. Thus the roles, which an individual is playing, are narrowed down. Old age is often considered a role-less period of life. According to Rosow (1978) very few roles, like senior citizen, retiree or grandparent are available to the elderly. Since roles contribute substantially to one's identity and self-esteem, the unavailability of viable roles can have negative effects on the self-image resulting in loss of self-esteem. The number of elderly is increasing in all the societies. This is mainly because of the increasing birth rate, the decreasing death rate in infancy, childhood, youth and middle age. The processes of urbanization and industrialization have led to the breakdown in the traditional care, which the family as a unit used to provide to the elderly. When children live in different places elder persons are left or choose to fend for themselves with diminishing physical, health and economic status. Their exclusion from traditional, social and familial roles of prestige and power or place them in a marginal position.

Therefore, it is worthwhile to study this phenomenon with a view to answering the following questions:

1. What transformations occur in the role and status system when the social subjects pass through adulthood to old age? (after the termination of occupational role)
2. In what ways do these changes affect the adaptability of elder persons?
3. Are there gender variations in the elderly?
4. What kind of impact does retirement have on their lives?

Methodology

The change in the social roles in old age has been studied in the present chapter in respect of women who have retired from government jobs. Three groups of women, i.e. school teachers (70), public servants (50), and professionals (30) were selected for the present study. They were 60–70 years old at the time of interview and were residents of Delhi. The social roles played by them before/after retirement were studied with the help of an interview schedule/scale. It seeks to explore if the termination of occupational role is a major transition in the life of women and to consider its course as a process of change and adaptation to new roles. Some roles cease to exist, others are added and some are modified to adapt to changing environment.

For the purpose of the present study, social roles are those roles which the women are expected to perform in their interpersonal relations with the family members, friends, neighbours and relatives. Their re-adaptation to new roles will depend on how they perceived their roles and developed strategies to cope with the changed social status in order to restore their social functioning.

Retirement age is considered that age after which the working women cease to be in active service at normal retirement age under a formal retirement system. This definition excludes all those working women who have taken voluntary retirement after putting in a minimum specified years of service.

For any government servant, retirement is inevitable. It is legitimately held that old age begins with retirement. It can be interpreted as the end of life or the beginning of a new phase depending upon the mental set-up and personality of the individual. It brings with it a feeling of uselessness, sense of non-entity causing depression of various kinds. The termination of occupational role brings about the "retirement crisis". It is considered as a stressful life event since a multiplicity of problems confront the individual. Cox (1984) describes that some of the problems of old age are lowering of income, loss of status, privilege and power that were associated with one's position in the occupational hierarchy, major reorganization of life's activities since the regular routine of the individual gets disrupted.

Thus retirement demands readjustment in the life of retirees in the living arrangement, financial status, health status, self-identity, self-worthy relationship with others and daily activities.

With the termination of the occupational role, there is change in the status of a woman perceived by herself as well as others surrounding her. She is categorized as a retired person, a free person who has nothing else to do or achieve in life. Unlike her male counterparts, she is welcomed in the household which has always been her primary domain. However, in most societies these women are categorized as "old" after retirement. The willingness on their part to accept the new roles is different from the willingness of those women who have stayed at home throughout their lives.

Thus, a question arises, how are the retired women able to perceive their new roles? They have to prepare themselves before retirement to accept the forthcoming roles. Sometimes the role player perceives a kind of conflict in her actual performance or in her ability to perform the various roles and the expectations of her "significant others". It is, therefore, important to study what kinds of roles our respondents play. How is their life affected after retirement? What do they feel about the meaningfulness of roles with their family members/ relations/others? Which are the roles that have terminated with retirement? Which are continuing? Which ones have emerged as new roles?

They all try to adjust to their retired status by modifying a routine role, changing one's attitude, filling a role void and making an attempt to assimilate their role in the total situation. Those who fail to develop a role balance in their personality continue to have poor life satisfaction (Zurcher, 1983). This creates a constant stress in the lives of retired women, which later becomes a cause for some physiological and psychological problems. Stress is built in the concept of role, which is conceived as the position a person occupies in a system, as defined by the expectations from others. Kahn et al. (1964) proposed three main role stresses: role conflict, role ambiguity and role overload. Pareek (1993) proposed ten organizational role stresses: self-role distance (SRD), inter-role distance (IRD), role stagnation (RS), role isolation (RI), role ambiguity (RA), role expectation conflict (REC), role overload (RO), role erosion (RE), resource inadequacy (RIA), and personal inadequacy (PIN). Research has been done on these role stresses, their nature and correlates. Bali (1999) in his article on well-being of the elderly illustrated with examples that life-satisfaction in retired women is affected sometimes by erosion in their roles, or an overload of roles and sometimes the elderly feel that they are isolated. All these factors are likely to lead to dissatisfaction among the elderly.

Impact of Retirement

The opinion of respondents was sought on the impact of retirement in major areas, which are likely to undergo change after retirement. These were: family life, living arrangement, financial status, health status, utilization of time gainfully, social network relationships, and overall life pattern. The data show that nearly 50 per cent of the respondents stated that their health status (48.7%), network relationships (54.7%) and ability to utilize time gainfully (48%) had deteriorated. For the remaining 50 per cent it either remained the same or got strengthened. But family life, living arrangement and financial status remained same in nearly 50 per cent of respondents. Thus, it is clear that the areas which are likely to deteriorate after retirement are health status, network relationship and ability to utilize their time gainfully. However, there was not much change in the family life, living arrangement and financial status of the retirement women (Figure 8.1).

Figure 8.1 : Impact of retirement on various aspects of lives of retirees

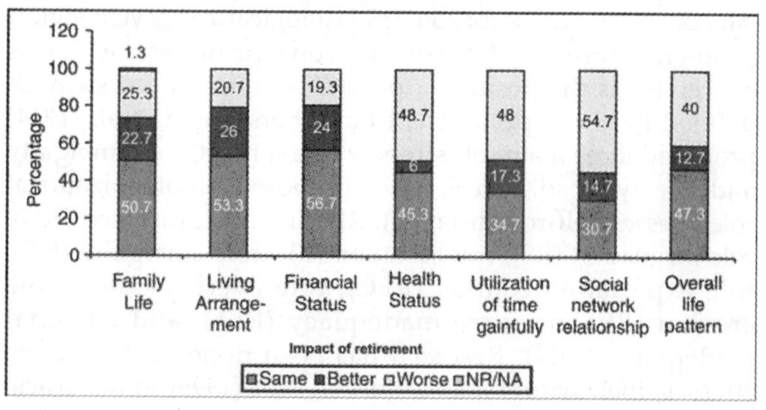

Opinion of Respondents on the Worth of Roles after Retirement

Amongst various role relationships with different persons, retired women felt that the role of a mother to children (35.3%), sister to sister (30%), and sister to brother (40%) and relative to relative (51.3%) deteriorated. Further, the role of a daughter/daughter-in-law was over in most of the cases. The two new roles which emerged with the onset of old age were those of grandmother and mother-in-law, neighbour (55%), homemaker (28.7%) and wife (33.7%).

TABLE 8.2 : Meaningfulness of Roles after Retirement

Role relation-ships	*Meaningfulness of Roles*						*Total*
	Same	*Regre-ssed*	*Expand-ed*	*Role over*	*New roles*	*NR/NA*	
Mother to children	20 (13.3%)	53 (35.3%)	21 (14.0%)	2 (1.3%)	-	54 (36.0%)	150 (100%)
Sister to sister	43 (28.7%)	45 (30.0%)	38 (25.3%)	6 (4.0)	-	18 (12.0%)	150 (100%)
Sister to brother	40 (26.7%)	60 (40.0%)	28 (18.7%)	7 (4.7)	-	15 (10.0%)	150 (100%)
Daughter to parents	7 (4.7%)	5 (3.3%)	10 (6.7%)	105 (70.0)	-	23 (15.3%)	150 (100%)
Grand-mother to grand-children	33 (22.0%)	15 (10.0%)	38 (25.3%)	1 (0.7)	9 (6.0%)	54 (36.0%)	150 (100%)
Wife	14 (9.3%)	21 (14.0%)	46 (30.7%)	33 (22.0%)	-	36 (24.0%)	150 (100%)
Daughter-in-law to parents-in-law	2 (1.3%)	7 (4.3%)	4 (2.7%)	82 (54.7%)	-	55 (36.7%)	150 (100%)
Mother-in-law to Daughter-in-law	28 (18.7%)	27 (18.0%)	19 (12.7%)	4 (2.7%)	4 (2.7%)	68 (45.3%)	150 (100%)
Mother-in-law to son-in-law	35 (23.3%)	25 (16.7%)	29 (19.3%)	4 (2.7%)	4 (2.7%)	53 (35.3%)	150 (100%)
Relative to relative	63 (42.0%)	77 (51.3%)	10 (6.7%)	-	-	-	150 (100%)
Friend to Friend	41 (27.3%)	74 (49.3%)	32 (21.3%)	3 (2.0%)	-	-	150 (100%)
Neighbour to neighbour	53 (35.3%)	41 (27.3%)	55 (36.7%)	-	-	1 (0.7%)	150 (100%)
As home member	65 (43.3%)	42 (28.0%)	43 (28.7%)	-	-	-	150 (100%)

Opinion of Respondents on Treatment meted out to them

The treatment meted out to respondents became relevant in the context of the opinion of respondents about the meaningfulness of roles being performed by them.

It is highly significant to note that although a considerable percentage of the respondents felt that their roles had become meaningless, they did not perceive the treatment meted out to them by their family members and other relatives had deteriorated. A majority of them felt that it had either remained the same or even became better. Only in nearly one-tenth of the respondents the treatment meted out to them had deteriorated (Table 8.3).

TABLE 8.3 : Treatment Meted out to Retirees after Retirement

Treatment meted to the respondent by	*Same*	*Better*	*Worse*	*NR/NA*	*New Relation-ship*	*Total*
Son(s)	42 (28.0%)	33 (22.0%)	19 (12.7%)	56 (37.3%)	-	150 (100%)
Daughter(s)	62 (41.3%)	33 (22.0%)	7 (4.7%)	48 (32.0%)	-	150 (100%)
Grand-Children	48 (32.0%)	24 (16.0%)	4 (2.7%)	53 (35.3%)	21 (14.0%)	150 (100%)
Sister(s)	83 (55.3%)	40 (26.7%)	9 (6.0%)	18 (12.0%)	-	150 (100%)
Brother(s)	97 (64.7%)	24 (16.0%)	11 (7.3%)	18 (12.0%)	-	150 (100%)
Husband	37 (24.7%)	34 (22.7%)	15 (10.0%)	64 (42.7%)	-	150 (100%)
Daughter-in-law	32 (21.3%)	20 (13.3%)	23 (15.3%)	70 (46.7%)	5 (3.3%)	150 (100%)
Son-in-law	76 (50.7%)	12 (8.0%)	8 (5.3%)	54 (36.0%)	-	150 (100%)
Relative	126 (84.0%)	13 (8.7%)	11 (7.3%)	-	-	150 (100%)
Friends	98 (65.3%)	32 (21.3%)	19 (12.7%)	1 (0.7%)	-	150 (100%)
Neighbours	106 (70.7%)	37 (24.7%)	6 (4.0%)	1 (0.7%)	-	150 (100%)
Servants	138 (92.0%)	1 (0.7%)	5 (3.3%)	6 (4.0%)	-	150 (100%)

In order to get an objective assessment of the change in roles being performed by the respondents after retirement, various role-related activities that are likely to be performed were identified and listed under each role area. The performance in each activity was classified on a five-point scale, i.e. "mostly", "often", "occasionally", "rarely" and "never". The weightage assigned to each choice ranged from 5 to 1. The respondent "most involved" in an activity was accorded maximum score, i.e. "5" and the respondent least involved got a score of "1". The respondents were asked to answer all the role-related activities before as well as after retirement on the basis of their degree of involvement. Finally overall involvement of one respondent in each area was calculated. This was done by adding up all the scores obtained by the respondents in various role-related activities. This score was taken for each area before as well as after retirement. Since the number of role-related activities under each role area was different, the average involvement of each respondent in all the role areas was calculated before as well as after retirement. Finally the student's t-test' was applied to study if difference between average performance in each role area, before/after retirement was statistically significant. The various role-related activities in different roles include writing letters, talking on phone, making visits, looking after day to day needs of the spouse/children, care-giving roles, extending emotional support, financial support, giving gifts to grandchildren.

It was found that the average involvement of all respondents while playing the roles of a wife, mother, sister (sister to sister, sister to brother), daughter-in-law, mother-in-law (mother-in-law to son-in-law), friend, relative and neighbour and home-maker was higher during the pre-retirement phase as compared to their post-retirement phase. In all roles except daughter-in-law and son-in-law there was a significant difference between mean values before and after retirement. The only three roles in which the average involvement of respondents was found to be low in pre-retirement period were those of the grandmother, daughter and mother-in-law (mother-in-law to daughter-in-law).

Relationship between Each Role and Total Roles before/after Retirement

It has been noted that role is a relational term. One plays a

TABLE 8.4 : Performance of Retirees in Role areas Before/ After Retirement (N =150)

Interaction with	*Before Retirement Mean*	*Standard Deviation*	*After Retirement Mean*	*Standard Deviation*	*t-value*
Children	2.91	1.54	2.18	1.25	11.17**
Sister	2.62	1.07	2.50	1.27	2.26*
Brother	2.41	1.05	2.24	1.19	3.17**
Parents	1.26	1.59	0.65	1.31	5.99**
Grand-children	1.41	1.53	1.84	1.59	4.49**
Husband	2.49	1.56	1.87	1.80	5.47**
Parents-in-law	1.10	1.60	0.34	1.00	6.63**
Daughter-in-law	1.35	1.53	1.46	1.53	1.59
Son-in-law	1.55	1.41	1.64	1.41	1.16
Relatives	2.35	0.53	2.24	0.52	3.59**
Friends	2.70	0.683	2.44	0.82	5.08**
Neighbours	2.47	0.62	2.67	0.86	3.78**
Home-maker	3.74	0.92	3.40	1.16	4.50**
Total roles	28.37	6.90	25.47	6.69	8..50**

*Significant at .05 level
** Significant at .01 level

role vis-à-vis another person. For example, a woman in the family plays the role of a daughter-in-law in relation to her mother-in-law. Mid-life women are workers, wives, mothers, daughters, sisters, home-makers, etc. In each sphere role partners surround them. All these roles are complementary. In each sphere it can be seen that the role expectations for each role are framed in accordance with the obligations over privileges.

The overall role of a woman is judged by how deeply she is involved in various roles individually and her overall role performance as an individual. The score of overall involvement of respondents in all role areas was taken to calculate correlation coefficient "r" between each role area with the total roles areas before as well as after retirement (Table 8.5).

TABLE 8.5 : Degree of Relationship Between Each Role and Total Roles Before/After Retirement

Relationship with	*Total Roles*	
	Before Retirement "r"	*After Retirement "r"*
Husband	.72**	.67**
Children	.72**	.68**
Sister	.02	.12
Brother	.30**	.39**
Parents	.24**	.27**
Parents-in-law	.63**	.44**
Daughter-in-law	.53**	.48**
Son-in-law	.55**	.63**
Grandchildren	.59**	.58**
Friends	.11	.32**
Relatives	.37**	.36**
Neighbour	.13	.34**
Home-maker	.13	.04

* significant at .05 level
**significant at .01 level

The data show that although the measure of correlation co-efficient went down after retirement, it remained statistically significant for all the roles being played by the respondents except those of the sister and the homemaker. However, correlation coefficient went up in the case of sister, daughter and mother-in-law to son-in-law, friends and neighbours.

Prioritization of Social Roles by the Retirees

The retirees were asked to answer all the role activities under each area. This had a limitation since their freedom was being restricted. Therefore, it was thought necessary to give them a choice and seek their opinion on three major roles being performed by them before as well as after retirement.

The main role being performed before retirement had been that of a wife, an employee and of a mother. After retirement, the women continued to play the role of a wife but the frequency of respondents continuing to play that role went down from 78 to 41. The second major role was that of a

Figure 8.2 : Most common social roles assumed by retirees (First priority)

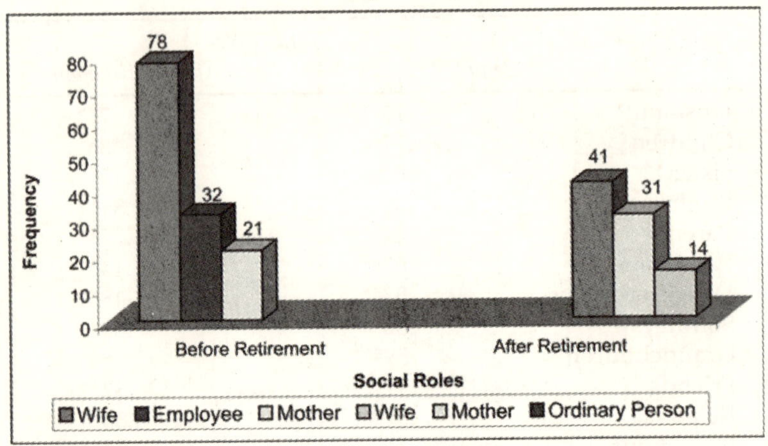

Figure 8.3 : Most common social roles assumed by retirees (Second priority)

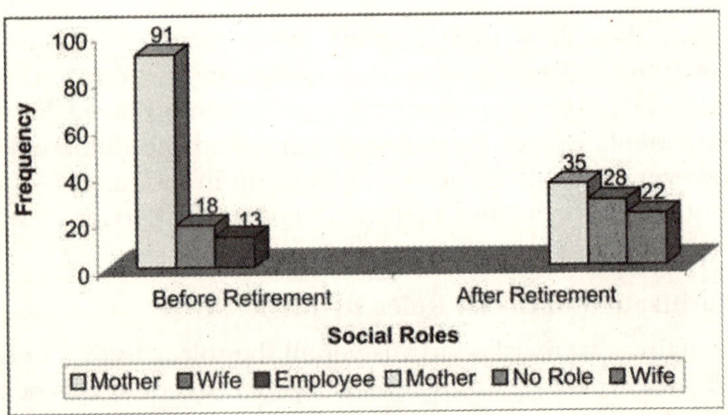

mother and the last one being that of an ordinary person. In the second priority also the roles revolved around that of mother, wife and employee though the sequence changed. However, it is highly significant to note that the frequency of respondents answering "no role" being played by them went up from 6 to 28 in the second priority and finally to 65 in the third priority after retirement. In the third priority the women

Figure 8.4 : Most common social roles assumed by retirees (Third priority)

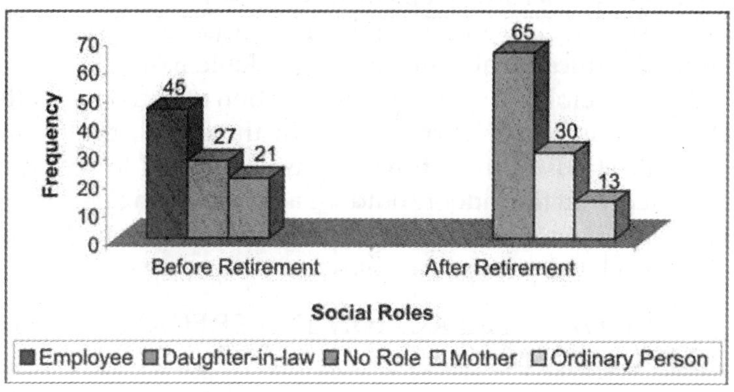

accorded it first rank. Figures 8.2, 8.3 and 8.4 depict the changes in the opinion of respondents.

From Figures 8.2, 8.3 and 8.4 it becomes clear that the roles of retirees revolve around that of wife, mother, mother-in-law, sister, employee, ordinary person and professional. They continue holding the same roles even after retirement but with little changes in the frequencies depending on the needs of the retirees. Further, a few new roles like grandmother, member of spiritual organization, etc. are added

TABLE 8.6 : Relationship of Social Roles with Social, Health, Economic Status, Indoor/Outdoor Activities, Age, Educational Status of the Female Retirees

Independent Variables	*Social Roles*
Age	- .29**
Social	.43**
Economic	.31**
Health	.17*
Indoor Activities	.45**
Outdoor Activities	.38**
Educational Status	.12

* Significant at 05 level

** Significant at 01 level

to their status and there is an increase in a few role areas.

The social roles being assumed by a retiree are not only dependent on her involvement in various role areas but also her present social, economic, health status, involvement in activities, educational status and age (Table 8.6).

Data in Table 8.6 show that assumption of social roles after retirement is highly correlated with the social, health and economic status of the retiree. It was also found to be highly correlated with the indoor/outdoor activities being performed after retirement. However, it was significant to note that age was not related with social roles.

DEGREE OF SATISFACTION IN PERFORMANCE OF VARIOUS ROLES

The degree of satisfaction in performance of various roles is also likely to vary from individual to individual since satisfaction is a relative term. The opinion of the respondents was sought on the degree of satisfaction in performing the sum total of various roles before as well as after retirement (Table 8.7).

TABLE 8.7 : Degree of Satisfaction in Performing sum total of Roles Before/After Retirement

Degree of satisfaction	*Before Retirement*	*After Retirement*
Fully Satisfied	50	88
Partially Satisfied	47	45
Dissatisfied	53	17
Total	150	150

The data show that amongst all the categories the degree of satisfaction in performing various roles after retirement is higher as compared to pre-retirement period. The respondents were asked to give reasons for their partial/total dissatisfaction. The reasons were overload, negative attitude of family members and incongenial relations with colleagues. Similarly, the reasons for being partially satisfied/dissatisfied after retirement were roles forced upon the retiree, death/sickness of spouse/child, overload or isolation.

CONCLUSION

After interviewing 150 women retirees from the workforce who were involved in different kind of occupations, it was found that the health, size of network and ability to utilize time gainfully deteriorates with the onset of retirement. However, their living arrangement, family life and financial status improved or remained the same. The social roles which were weak after retirement include role of a mother, sister, friend and relative. It declined after retirement whereas the remaining roles (grandmother, mother-in-law, neighbour and homemaker) gained momentum after retirement. Although some roles did show deterioration after retirement, the retirees do not feel that the treatment meted out to them by the family members and other relatives also goes down. It was the same/ better in all the cases. The involvement of respondents in all the role areas is more before retirement and the difference between the various roles performed before/after retirement was found to be statistically significant except that of daughter-in-law and son-in-law. From the data, it is inferred that social roles are positively correlated with social, economic and health status of the retiree. They are also related with indoor/ outdoor activities. The two variables which were not found to be related with social roles included "education" and "age".

The three roles in which the average involvement of respondents was found to be low in pre-retirement period were those of grandmother, daughter-in-law and mother-in-law.

It is interesting to note that when the retirees were asked to prioritize their roles before/after retirement, it was found that the main role in first priority was that of wife, employee and mother before retirement but after retirement the category of 'no role' showed a significant increase. Similarly the role of mother/wife also went down after retirement.

Further, the activities which take precedence in later years were making phone calls, nurturance/care-giver, extending emotional support and spending time with grandchildren. The increase in the frequency of exchanging gifts took place only with children and grandchildren otherwise it declined after retirement.

Thus, it can be concluded that social roles are never static. The roles a person assumes and plays depend on various factors such as age, mental status, physical condition, socio-economic and cultural background. These roles are different for different life phases. There is a major transition in roles from adulthood to old age. Amongst the elderly also, the roles played by persons show gender-wise/occupation-wise variation. With the termination of occupational role of women, the expectation of family/society from the retirees are same as from housewives. But the adaptation to these emerging roles varies in both the groups. The former have been in employment throughout their lives as a result of which they feel threatened in losing the power of making decisions and other benefits enjoyed by them throughout their life. With the end of occupational role, the category of 'no role' takes precedence over other roles. It is the dominating role which affects the entire physical, psychological, emotional and social life of retired women.

REFERENCES

Bali, A.P. (1999). Well being of the elderly, *Social Change*, March–June, 29(1,2), 64–76.

Brim, O.G. and Wheeler, S. (1966). Socialization after Childhood, New York: John Wiley.

Cox, H. (1984). Later Life: The Realities of Aging, New Jersey: Prentice Hall Inc.

Erikson, E.H. (1963). Childhood and Society (2nd ed.), New York: Norton.

Havighurst, R.J. (1972). Life Style and Leisure Patterns: Their evolution through the life cycle. International Course in Social Gerontology, 3, Proceedings, 35–48.

Heiss, J. (1981). Social Roles. In M. Rosenberg and R.H. Turner (eds.), Social Psychology Sociological Perspective, New York: Basic Books.

Hurlock, E.B. (1980). Developmental Psychology: A life span approach (5th ed.), New York: McGraw-Hill.

Kahn, R.L., Donald, M.W., Robert, P., Quinn, J., Diedrick S. and Rosehthai, R.A. (1964). Organizational Stress, Studies in Role Conflict and Ambiguity, New York: John Wiley.

Linton, R. (1968). The cultural background of personality, London: Routledge and Kegan.

Merton, R.K. (1957). The role set, *British Journal of Sociology*, 8 June, 106–120.

Sneugarten, B. and Datan, N. Sociological perspectives on the life cycle. In Paul Baltes and K. Warner. (1973). Schaie (ed.), Life Span Developmental Psychology: *Personality and Socialization*, New York: Academic Press, pp. 53–69.

Pareek, U. (1993). Role stress and coping: A framework in Pareek, U. and Pestonjee, D.M. (eds.) Studies in organizational role stress and coping, Jaipur, Rawat Publications, pp. 1–40.

Rosow, I.S. (1976). and Role change through the life span. In R.H. Binstock and E. Shanas (eds.) Handbook of Aging and the social sciences, New York: Van Nostrand Reinhold Company.

Zurcher, A.L. (1983). Social Roles: Conformity, conflict and creativity, Beverly Hills: Sage Publications.

Chapter 9

Gender Issues in HIV/AIDS

Neeti Malhotra

According to one estimate, there are 600,000 people with AIDS and 4.58 million infected with HIV in India. As per the latest estimates of National AIDS Control Organization (NACO), 25% of the 3.97 million people living with HIV/AIDS in India are women. This contributes to a further rise in paediatric AIDS. Figures from UNAIDS state that 0.8% of the total adult population (15–49 years) in India is living with HIV or AIDS out of which 1.5 million are women in the age group 15–24 years. Variation thus exists in reported epidemiological data from different sources. However, there is a general consensus that worldwide approximately as many women as men suffer from HIV. Yet the implications of the condition are severely different for women compared to men. Schneider (1992) makes four general sociological observations concerning HIV/AIDS and elaborates how, besides race and class, gender is the most determinant of a person's health status or his or her degree of well being. Gender (apart from race and class) will affect perceptions of health and illness, kinds and availability of care, modes of delivery, anticipated illnesses and discourse and interaction patterns of doctor-patient relationships. Social relations on gender emerge from and result in inequalities of social and political power and control over labour, resources and services. Also, gender relations influence the experiences of people with AIDS, community and political reactions, the nature of institutional practice and the dynamics of change in society. Thus it is accepted that AIDS as a biological and medical phenomenon of the late twentieth century, has and will continue to affect gender relations.

Marked differences can be cited in the impact of AIDS on women vis-à-vis men. Some of these result from the biological differences in sex between men and women. Women become more susceptible to HIV infection during a heterosexual intercourse due to:

- the greater area of mucous membrane exposed during sex in women than in men,
- the greater quantity of fluids transferred from men to women,
- the higher viral content of male sexual fluids,
- the microtears that can occur in vaginal (or rectal) tissue from sexual penetration. Younger women may be even more susceptible to infection (WHO, 2004). Scientific studies suggest (in cases where there are no untreated sexually transmitted diseases a STDs) that a man with HIV has a one in 500 chance of passing HIV to his partner in a single act of vaginal intercourse. In the same circumstance the chances for a woman to infect a man are about one in 1000.

However, socially defined gender differences are comparatively more responsible for the imbalances in the proportion of impact of HIV suffered by women. Gender can be defined as an array of societal beliefs, norms, customs and practices that define 'masculine' and 'feminine' attributes and behaviours. Being a social construct, gender differentiates the role, power, responsibilities and obligations of women from that of men in society (WHO, 2002). In several societies, gender norms, for example, allow men to have more sexual partners than women and encourage older men to have sexual relations with younger women. Men need to take risks and therefore have multiple partners. For instance, there is a belief among truckers in India that sexual release is essential after driving every 400 km to release the tension (VSO,2003). In some African countries, there is a phenomenon of 'sugar daddies' where older men have sexual relations with younger girls in the belief that younger girls are not infected. In conjunction with the biological factors and places where heterosexual transmission is the main mode of HIV infection (as in the case of India), infection rates among younger women can be much higher compared to younger men. Entrenched beliefs in society mean that generally women are less powerful to decide with whom, when and how they have sex. As per women's organizations, most of the women living with HIV/AIDS in India acquired the infection through their husbands (VSO, 2003).

Besides being a social construct, gender is also a culture-specific construct. So, there is a significant difference between what a woman or a man can or cannot do in one culture as compared to another. However, in a fairly consistent way it is found that there is a distinct difference between women's and men's roles, access to productive resources and decision-making authority. Women comparatively have less access to and control over productive resources than men creating an unequal balance of power that favours men. Gender gaps between men and women in literacy, school enrolment, labour force participation, land ownership and access to credit testify to this imbalance in power (UNIFEM, 2000). This inequity also translates into differences in male and female sexuality. In the case of girls, patriarchy imposes a constraint as sexuality becomes a limiting factor in girls' lives (Greene, 1997). Forming the core of gender ideology in India are the concepts of *izzat* and *sharam* (i.e. honour and shame) which define the way a girl should conduct herself as soon as she reaches puberty (Bhattacharjee, 2004). In fact, in most societies in the world, virginity, chastity, motherhood, moral superiority and obedience are deemed to be the key virtues of an ideal woman. Thus, the dominant ideology of femininity casts women in a subordinate, dependent and passive position. Because of this dominant world view of women as subservient, HIV/AIDS programmes also largely view women merely as vectors of the infection. HIV interventions are disease or merely as bearers of unborn children. The design of HIV interventions is therefore influenced by this ideology and are likely to be counterproductive. Women lack direct control over the preventive remedy offered to them by public health, i.e. the condom—that requires active participation of male partners (Wermuth et al., 1992). There is talk of a female condom being available soon but the questions of its affordability and access persist (Mane, 20 July 2004, *Times of India*) Freedom of choice without the economic means to exercise it is quite meaningless.

Gender mores dictate that women should be ignorant and passive about sex. Lack of knowledge and incomplete knowledge also leads to fears and myths about condom use (Rao Gupta and Weiss, 1993). The dominant ideology of masculinity on the other hand characterizes men as aggressive, dominant and independent. Thus men remain ignorant because they are supposed to know everything about sex. As a result, many men have erroneous information about sexual and reproductive health (UNAIDS, 1999). Gender norms also create pressures on them to take risks and prove their manhood by having sex with multiple partners (Silberschmidt, 2001).

Women are often socially, economically and physically more vulnerable than men. It is difficult to imagine how safer sex can be negotiated when the cultural taboo against sexual talk continues to exist. Women encounter interactional or practical difficulties when they introduce condoms into a sexual scene or talk about changing sexual practice (Schnieder, 1992). Research suggests that women occasionally experience violence by their partners when they try to raise the issue of safer sex and the use of condoms. So fear of violence exacerbates the incidence of HIV infection in women. Additionally, fear of stigma and abandonment can dissuade women from learning about their HIV status or if they do learn it from sharing it with their partners. It can also have a detrimental effect on HIV control, treatment and prevention of mother to child transmission programmes (WHO, 2004).

These socially determined gender roles also affect access to health services including those for HIV/AIDS. Traditionally, more resources are allocated for men and boys. Conditioned to perform a sacrificial role, women give priority to their husband's or children's health and do not seek medical attention till they are seriously ill. Care organizations in India say that generally only 25% of the hospital beds are taken by women as men are traditionally given priority for treatment given their role as breadwinners. Use of services are also limited for women because of constraints on their mobility, practices such as the 'purdah' and non-availability of women-friendly medical care, i.e. facilities which ensure privacy or seclusion and in some cases even emotional support for women to feel comfortable to use the service. Economic factors also significantly determine whether or not women will access health care services. Besides payment of services, a woman is also constrained by money for transportation, high opportunity cost for lost time, large workloads (amounting on an average to 10–16 hours a day worldwide) and engagement in insecure jobs which make it difficult for them to take time off to access health care. Equal access to treatment (including anti-retroviral drugs), care and prevention information is vital to slowing down the impact of AIDS.

In this scenario, experiences from countries where free and universal access to anti-retroviral therapy is allowed also throws a special insight. Is free service the answer? It seems not. In Brazil, noticeable gender differences were found in the seeking and use of free services. Voluntary testing and counselling is offered in pre-natal clinics. The attitudes of health workers is also a limitation as they treat infected women as intravenous drug users or prostitutes. Also, women are often not diagnosed till the late stages of infection as they typically don't use the clinics until late pregnancy (WHO, 2002). Therefore gender-related factors increase a woman's economic vulnerability, making her more susceptible to HIV, restricting access to services and information thereby increasing morbidity.

Ironically, the reverse does not make men better health care seekers. Notions of masculinity contribute to making the socialization of men as self-reliant and invulnerable. So not only do such notions encourage risk taking (through unsafe sex or drugs) as such behaviour defines 'real' men but also deters men from seeking health care. Another reason that keeps men away from accessing HIV/AIDS information and services is that often these services are provided in prenatal, family planning or child health clinics which are simply not designed to reach men or meet their needs. Men are thus less likely to be fully informed about HIV/AIDS prevention, care and support and treatment options (Mane and Aggleton, 2001), thereby reducing men's ability to protect themselves or cope with AIDS.

Notions of masculinity emphasise sexual domination of women as the defining characteristic of manhood. Such an overpowering notion of male sexuality, quite obviously disregards alternate sexuality and thus leads to homophobia and stigmatization of men who have sex with men. This in turn coerces men who have sex with men to keep their sexual preference a secret and deny their sexual risk, hence increasing their own risk as well as that of their partners, whether male or female.

ADOLESCENTS AND YOUTH

The situation of adolescents and youth in the context of HIV/AIDS is an example of how gender and age intersect to determine the distribution of power in society. Therefore, typically younger members of a society have lesser power than older people and younger girls have lesser power (and lesser control over their bodies) than younger boys/men. Adolescence is a stage in which growing girls and boys often go through a period of confusion trying to reconcile the conflict between their own sexual curiosity and urges on one side and the societal/familial expectations from them on the other side. There are significant differences in socialization of young boys and girls. An adolescent's choice of time use, type of education, mobility, access to information and even decision-making responsibility within home is determined by his/her gender. Young boys thus end up getting 'sexual privileges' where sex is accepted as a 'necessity' for them whereas 'a number of responsibilities are assigned to young women—

including safeguarding her virginity, responsibility of birth control and insistence that ignorance about sex is the best protection from sexual interactions.

VIOLENCE AGAINST WOMEN

Violence against women is another disturbing outcome of this societal emphasis on physical and sexual domination of women being essential for being 'manly'. According to studies conducted all over the world, 10 to over 50% of women report physical assault by an intimate partner of which one-third to half also report sexual coercion (Heise & Elias, 1995). HIV transmission becomes even more likely in the case of forced sex (experienced by many more women than men) since it may result in more trauma and vaginal tearing or lacerations (Maman et al., 2000). Research conducted in several countries including India has found that violence against women contributes both directly and indirectly to women's vulnerability to HIV. Fear of violence or abandonment also deters women from asking questions about fidelity or talking about condom use. This fear has also been found to be a barrier in reducing perinatal transmission of HIV, as women refuse HIV testing or don't return for results.

MOTHERHOOD AND HIV/AIDS

In many societies, another feminine ideal is motherhood, which poses a barrier in HIV risk reduction as use of condoms or non-penetrative sex prevents conception. In some societies, children provide women a social identity and guarantee them some status in kinship groups, while in others children are a means of getting assured economic support from the fathers (UNAIDS, 1999). Translating all these factors into programmatic realities, where the emphasis is on preventing transmission to the unborn child, the woman may lose her right to be informed and make a choice about what is best for her and her child by opting to go in for HIV testing, or an intervention to prevent mother to child transmission (MTCT) or abortion. These programmes also exclude the men, once again making it only the woman's responsibility.

Some HIV/AIDS programmes also discourage breastfeeding, which becomes a cause for stigma for women. Breastfeeding is seen as an integral part of the ideal of motherhood and in many places women who do not breastfeed are seen as bad mothers or treated as handicapped (Rao Gupta, 2000).

Burden of care

Apart from the personal risk of infection, women shoulder another big burden of AIDS. Majority of the caretaking for HIV-positive family members or those negatively affected by the disease such as AIDS orphans, falls on the women. Older women are being more burdened as they have to take care of their grandchildren after their own children have died of AIDS. There is often no material or psychological support available to these women. Gender norms also influence men's lack of involvement in the caring responsibilities which often means that they are distanced from the gravity of the situation and continue to perpetuate the gender stereotypes.

LOWER ECONOMIC STATUS AND VULNERABILITY TO HIV

There is a direct link between women's low economic status and their vulnerability and exposure to HIV. Poverty is the biggest cause of women bartering sex for economic gain or survival. Research also shows that women who enter sexual relationships due to economic reasons have more chances of getting syphilis or HIV. Poverty also prevents women from negotiating safer sex or opting out of a risky relationship due to fear of destitution or abandonment (Weiss and Rao Gupta, 1998). It has been shown that women in high-risk relationships perceive the short-term costs of leaving the relationship much higher than the potential long-term health costs. For those who are economically disadvantaged (either men or women), lack of access to information and knowledge is also very real. Studies have shown that knowledge of HIV/AIDS prevention is much higher among the economically advantaged than among those who are less so (Gwatkin and Deveshwar-Bahl, 2001).

MIGRATION

Lack of employment opportunities and poverty force both men and women to migrate in search of work. This disrupts stable social and familial relationships. Separation from the partner can lead to both men and women forming new sexual networks. In the case of seasonal migration, when men return home to their community of origin, their female partners (who are left behind) are very vulnerable. It has been found that their wives of long-term sexual partners are unable to insist on condom use when the men have returned after so long working to send money at home. For the men, it is likely that they had sexual relations while being away from home simply due to a basic sexual urge, or for economic gain or security.

COPING WITH HIV/AIDS

Just as there are significantly different ways in which men and women experience poverty, research has shown that women are generally more vulnerable to the consequences of AIDS' morbidity and mortality. The differential response begins soon after a positive HIV diagnosis. Women are often subjected to violence when they are tested positive antenatally. When men are diagnosed positive, women are mostly blamed for the infection and subjected to violence, abandonment or property grabbing. According to Positive Women's Network, India, women living with HIV/AIDS in India (particularly widows) are very vulnerable to property theft from their relatives (VSO, 2003).

While education does empower, in matters of sexuality and fertility, it has been found that even educated women are not equipped to make an informed choice. Information and knowledge about reproductive health, sexual development during adolescence, HIV/AIDS and drug abuse are not covered in the school curriculum or even at college.

Rising incidence of AIDS has compelled the introduction of information dissemination on closeted subjects like puberty and sexual changes to adolescent boys and girls. Experience has shown that information about the body not only leads to better hygienic and nutritional practices by teenagers but also brings about a positive change in their concepts of dignity, relationships and aspirations. Sex education has been found to have a differential impact on boys and girls. Where for boys it is simply information on bodily changes and contraception, for girls it has also meant confidence building, freedom of movement and career aspirations. However, a study of sex education programmes under AIDS prevention reveals that these programmes do not discuss condom promotion or son preference with unmarried boys and girls. Subjects such as sexuality are obliquely addressed. Even in a major education programme like the University Talk AIDS of the Government of India, sexuality was not dealt with. Among the listed factors that lead youth to high risk situations, the words 'sex' and 'sexuality' do not occur even once among the seven points laid down (Bhattacharjee, 2004). As Dr Nafis Sadik, executive director UNFPA comments, "Across South Asia, there is no real sex education. And health services outside marriage are practically nil." (quoted in Bhattacharjee 2004, p. 227) Experts believe that a change in the political mindset will be needed to bring about the essential shift. On the other hand, young people express a huge need for sex education and are certain that education about sex and protective methods will not lead to promiscuity (Malhotra, 2002). The other aspect of all this is that knowledge alone is not enough and the real problem is that women do not have any control over their bodies—it is the patriarchal structure that rules over it. In fact knowledge without empowerment can be more detrimental to girls than no knowledge at all.

APPROACHES TO ADDRESS GENDER IN HIV/AIDS

In many ways, HIV/AIDS is a unique biopsychosociological phenomenon, which has thrown up a myriad moral, ethical, legal and human rights issues on a scale not witnessed before. Looking at HIV/AIDS through the gender lens adds another dimension to this complexity. Programme managers and policy makers need to work under guidelines to integrate gender issues into HIV/AIDS programming.

A review of programmatic responses to address gender

issues in HIV/AIDS has shown that there is a continuum of approaches, which range from harmful to empowering. Interventions, which reinforce damaging gender·sexual stereotypes, perpetuate the epidemic either directly or indirectly. Gender-sensitive intervention appreciated the differences between the needs of men and women and finds ways to meet those needs differently. A step up are gender transformative interventions which not only recognise the distinctions between the needs of men and women but also create conditions by which women and men can examine the damaging aspects of gender norms and experiment with new behaviours to create more equitable roles and relationships. At the end of the continuum are structural interventions, which go beyond health interventions to reduce gender inequalities through empowering women and girls by increasing their access to economic and social resources. A 1999 review of HIV/AIDS programmatic activities which attempted to address gender dimensions in prevention, care, treatment and social support by UNAIDS concluded that albeit on a limited scale, HIV/AIDS programmes that address gender equality as a central goal maximize their overall effectiveness (WHO, 2002).

There are many layers of masculinity and femininity, which vary according to social class, ethnicity, sexuality and age. Through social interaction, it is possible to bring about modifications in the construction of gender identities, which can promote more equitable gender relationship and safer sex. Gender issues should thus be addressed and analyzed in all aspects of planning, implementation, monitoring and evaluation of policies, programmes, projects and research. Technical/substantive aspects of gender integration refer to specific approaches and strategies used to address gender differences. In its most basic way, what a gendered response to AIDS demands is the elimination of those stereotypes which inhibit or curtail a woman's or man's ability to benefit from HIV/AIDS intervention. For instance, HIV/AIDS preventive messages which show women as only 'victims' (and thereby powerless) or 'repositories' or 'carriers of the disease'.

Programming should be needs based in that when the needs of men and women are different, there should be different programmes. But equally important are cases where the needs of women and men are the same, the services should not treat them differently. One such example is that of information of perinatal transmission of HIV which is often given only to women thereby: *(i)* discouraging parenting as a joint responsibility of both mother and father *(ii)* reinforcing the stereotype of women as 'vectors' of the disease *(iii)* making it more likely for men to block through female partners use of mother to child transmission prevention services as they are not fully conversant with its benefits. It is important therefore to design interventions based on information and good understanding of how gender constructs impact the vulnerability of both men and women to HIV/AIDS.

REFERENCES

Bhattacharjee, S. (2004). The Politics of Silence : Introducing sex education in India In Mohan Rao (ed.) *The Unheard Scream,* Zubaan, New Delhi.

Greene, M.E. (1997). Watering the Neighbour's Garden: Investing in Adolescent Girls in India, South and East Asia Regional Paper No.7, Population Council, New Delhi.

Gwatkin, D.R. and Deveshwar-Bahl, G. (2001). Inequalities in Knowledge of HIV/AIDS Prevention: An overview of socio-economic and gender differentials in developing countries. Unpublished draft.

Heise, L. and Elias, C. (1995). Transforming AIDS prevention to meet women's needs: a focus on developing countries. *Social Science and Medicine,* 40(7): 933–943.

Malhotra, N. (2002). Role of Communication in AIDS Prevention, Ph.D Thesis submitted to the Department of Social Work, Jamia Millia Islamia, New Delhi.

Maman, S., Campbell, J. et al. (2000). The Intersections of HIV and Violence: Directions for future Research and Interventions. *Social Science and Medicine,* 50: 459–487.

Mane, P. and Aggleton, P. (2001). Gender and HIV/AIDS: What do men have to do with it? *Current Sociology,* 49 (6): 23–37.

Gupta, G.R. and Weiss, E. (1993). Women and AIDS: "Developing a

New Health Strategy". Washington DC, International Centre for Research on Women.

Gupta, G.R. (2000). Gender, Sexuality and HIV/AIDS: The What, the Why, and the How (Plenary Address) XIII Conference on HIV/AIDS, Durban, South Africa.

Schnieder, B. (1992). AIDS and Class, Gender and Race Relations In Joan Huber and Beth E Schnieder (eds.) *The Social Context of AIDS,* American Sociological Association Presidential Series, Newbury Park : Sage.

Silberschmidt, M. (2001). Disempowerment of Men in Rural and Urban East Africa: Implications for male identity and sexual behaviour. World Development, 29(4): 657–671.

Times of India, 20 July 2004, *Soft Targets* (Purnima Mane in an interview to Bachi Karkaria).

Ellen, W. and Gupta, G.R. (1998). Bridging the Gap: Addressing Gender and Sexuality in HIV prevention. Washington, DC, International Centre for Research on Women.

Ellen, W. et al. (1996). Vulnerability and Opportunity: Adolescents and HIV/AIDS in the Developing World. Washington, DC, International Centre for Research on Women.

Wermuth, L. et al. (1992). Women don't wear Condoms: AIDS risk among sexual partners of IV Drug users In Joan Huber and Beth E Schnieder (ed.) The Social Context of AIDS, American Sociological Association Presidential Series, Newbury Park: Sage.

UNIFEM. (2000). Progress of the World's women 2000: Trends and Statistics. New York, United Nations Publication.

UNAIDS. (1999). Gender and HIV/AIDS: Taking stock of research and programmes. Geneva, UNAIDS.

Voluntary Services Overseas. (2003). Gendering AIDS: Women, men, empowerment, mobilisation, VSO AIDS Agenda, October 2003.

World Health Organization. (2002). Integrating Gender into HIV/AIDS Programmes, Expert Consultation, 3–5 June 2002, Geneva.

World Health Organization. (2004). Gender and Women's Health—Gender and HIV/AIDS. http://www.who.int/gender/hiv_aids/en/.

World Health Organization. (2004). Violence against women and HIV/AIDS (http://www.who.int/gender/violence/vawandhiv/en/)

Chapter 10

HIV/AIDS : A Study of Knowledge, Attitudes, Gender Equality and Professional Preparation among Social Work Students in India

Paul Sachdev

Since the first few cases of AIDS were detected in 1986 among female sex workers in Chennai and a short time later in Bombay (New Mumbai), the HIV virus has continued its devastating march across India, with more infections and deaths. There were an estimated 4.6 million HIV-infected individuals at the end of 2002, a significant leap from the 2001 figure of 3.97 million. This gives India the status of having the second highest number of infections in the world after South Africa (*India Today*, 27 July 2003; UNAIDS, 2000). The pandemic is spreading at twice the rate from urban to rural population, mainly through heterosexual transmission which accounts for almost 80 per cent (International AIDS conference, Durban, July 2000). Six states (i.e., Andhra Pradesh, Karnataka, Maharashtra, Manipur, Nagaland and Tamil Nadu) are particularly the worst hit. Because of poor or inadequate health infrastructures, uneven coordination between local and national levels and among non-government organizations (NGOs), the march of the deadly virus is not likely to be halted (Potts and Walsh, 2003). It is projected that the virus will infect 25 million people by the year 2010 making India as the future AIDS capital of the world (Agency France-Presse/Yahoo! News, 25 July, 2003;

Center for Strategic and International Studies, Washington cited in AIDS-India e-Forum, 18 November, 2003; National Intelligence Council, September 2002; National AIDS Control Organization (NACO) 2000; Nath, 2000).

Initially, the government and the health care providers dismissed it as a prostitute's disease. The notion of "otherness", that is by associating HIV/AIDS with the Western countries and with women who are promiscuous, irresponsible and sinful (i.e. the prostitutes), made it convenient for the government and health officials to cognitively distance themselves from the disease and this group of women who were afflicted. It was not until the deadly virus made its way from sex workers and their clients on to college campuses and into the bedrooms of married monogamous wives that government and health officials started to panic. Women are being infected with the HIV virus at higher rates than men (Gangakhedkar et al., 1997). According to the Alan Guttmacher Institute, New York the ratio of women to men infected with AIDS was 1 to 7 in 1992; by the year 2002, it approached one to one (Dube, 2000). Women's social subordination and unequal power relations to men are key determinants in their vulnerability to HIV/AIDS. Women who face the greatest risk are those with the least control, especially in an intimate heterosexual encounter, and are generally poor and uneducated women. Three-quarters of women have been infected within marriage by their HIV-positive husbands, even if they knew their husbands were infected. (*The Hindu*, 29 January 2004; Peter Piot, head of the UNAIDS at the International Conference of South Asian Parliamentarians in N. Delhi, 1–2 August, 2003). Since women have a larger mucosa surface exposed during sexual intercourse, it is easier for women to become infected than men. Studies show that the risk of women contracting HIV from men is 10 to 18 times greater than the risk of men getting the virus from women which suggests that women are often the victims and not the cause (UNIFEM, 2003).

With the revelation that transmission of the human immunodeficiency virus (HIV) largely takes place in India through heterosexual routes, the early high-risk groups identified as sex workers, homosexuals and intravenous drug users were then expanded to include young adults, aged 16–25. Young people account for nearly half of all new HIV/AIDS infections. (Bharat, 1996; National AIDS Control Organization, 1994: 16; UNICEF, 2003) It is in this context that young adults, as a special category, emerged and gained currency in studies of knowledge and attitudes regarding HIV/AIDS, and their sexual behaviour. The few recent studies on these young people (mostly college students) in India reveal an increased heterosexual activity which usually takes place with minimal or non-use of condoms making them at increased risk of HIV infection. (Abraham, 2001; Aggrawal et al., 2000; Amalraj et al., 1995; Awasthi, et al. 2000; Bourdier, 1998; Collumbien et al., 2001; Dube, 2000; FPAI, 1993; India Today Marg-Poll, 1994; Kumar et al., 1997; Koziara et al, 1994; Mathai et al., 1997; Melkote & Goswami, 2000; Nath, 2000; Sachdev, 1994; Sachdev, 1997; Selvan et al., 2001; Sharma & Sharma, 1996; Solomon et al., 1998; Watsa,1990). Nationally, barely more than 3% of sexually active people regularly use condoms. Even then, it is mainly to prevent conception rather than for protection against HIV and other sexually transmitted diseases (Farah, 2002, in National AIDS Control Organization News Bulletin, January 2002; UNAIDS News, January 2002). Recognizing that the pandemic continues to shift toward young men and women, some state governments, like West Bengal, have made it mandatory for young people to get tested for HIV infection prior to their wedding. The National AIDS Control Organization (NACO), too, has renewed its commitment toward increasing awareness and AIDS education among youth (*India Today*, 27 July 2003). The assumption is that correct information about the mode of transmission will lead to behaviour change in favour of abstinence or safer sex practices and develop a positive attitude towards people with HIV/AIDS (PWHA). There is some evidence that AIDS awareness programmes have not shown significant success in behaviour change among young people or made them more aware of the risk from the disease. For example, Dube (2000), a member of the World Bank team which reviewed the government's performance, observed: "The government commitment had faltered dangerously when it came to implementing these fine plans, especially the sexuality-related programmes" (p. 91).

Studies have shown that young people have a feeling of invulnerability and are not concerned about HIV/AIDS despite their knowledge of the risk (Anderson et al., 1990; Gray and Saracino,1991; Michael et al., 1994; Moore and Rosenthal, 1991, 1993; Richard and van der Pligt, 1991; Romer et al., 1994; Rotheram-Bonus et al., 1995; Sachdev, 1993; Slonim-Nevo et al., 1991). According to one recent research study in the state of Tamil Nadu only 35% of university students believed they were at risk of HIV (UNAIDS News, January 2002). Despite massive campaigns by NACO and 735 NGOs, aimed at creating community awareness, there is strong evidence that widespread ignorance about the disease and prejudice against PWHA persists among students in high schools and colleges as well as the general public (Marcelo, 2003; *Times News Network*, 13 November 2003: 2). To evaluate the impact of an awareness programme in Jharkhand, one of the high HIV prevalence areas, a recent study was conducted by the Centre for Social Research. The sample included 299 college students and a sample from general public. It found that only half of the respondents knew that AIDS could be prevented and only one in five knew that AIDS was incurable. (*Times News Network*, 13 November 2003). Having reviewed the studies conducted in India on AIDS awareness, attitudes and perception of risk, NACO concluded that: (*i*) most individuals do not have accurate and complete information on HIV/AIDS; (*ii*) the link between STDs and AIDS is not clear to most people, and (*iii*) there is a belief that HIV transmission and AIDS are found among limited groups such as foreigners, homosexuals, sex workers and drug users (NACO, 1997–98: 51).

Experience with infectious diseases has shown that perception and meaning associated with the disease (e.g., moral connotation, etiology of the disease being associated with prostitutes, gay people, intravenous drug users and their life style) profoundly influence attitudes toward people infected and affected by the disease and thus have a significant impact on the patient care (Temoshok et al., 1987). News reports indicate that a large majority of the general public, including health care professionals, hold negative and adverse attitudes toward HIV/AIDS patients who are subjected to discrimination and humiliation or even refused treatment (AIDS-India e-Forum, 20 & 22 November, 2003; Singh and Maliya, 1994; *The Hindu, Madurai Edition,* 19 July 2003). On 3 October 2003, Gita Bhawan Hospital in Indore issued a policy statement advising doctors to not provide treatment to HIV positive patients (*The Hindustan Times,* 15 October 2003. More recently, a widow, in the State of Andhra Pradesh, who had contracted the virus from her husband was stoned to death by her relatives and fellow villagers (*The Hindu, Madurai Edition* 19 July 2003). There are some reports that children of HIV parents have been denied regular schooling and an HIV-positive soldier was dismissed from the army (Associated Free Press, 26 October 2003). A few studies have suggested a positive relationship between accurate information about the disease and empathic attitude toward the infected person, (Ambati et al., 1997; Gray and Saracino, 1991; Ismail et al., 1995; Melkote and Goswami, 2000; Silberman, 1991; Weiner and Siegel, 1990). However, there are other researchers whose findings failed to agree with this claim (Owens, 1992; Walter et al., 1992). Some studies have suggested that in addition to fear of contagion, discomfort in working with AIDS patients may be associated with underlying anxiety about homosexuality. There is evidence that negative attitudes toward homosexuals are quite prevalent among health care professionals and social workers (Gillman,1991; Kelly et al., 1987; Reed et al., 1984; Van Servellen et al., 1988; Weiner and Siegel, 1990; Young, 1988). In spite of the reports confirming that HIV infection in India has largely spread through heterosexual means, AIDS continues to be cast in the public's mind as a sexually transmitted gay disease. The Indian Penal Code, under section 377, criminalizes homosexual act between two adults, though consensual, which may further reinforce prejudicial attitudes among the public and professionals.

As the AIDS crisis deepens in India and the number of infected women, men and children escalate, the role of social workers as part of the health care team becomes increasingly vital. Social workers are expected to provide AIDS education, counselling and promoting HIV-risk reduction behaviour in addition to assisting patients to cope with their disease and obtain treatment. Social workers whose work brings them in close contact with HIV-positive people are required to assist their families and the community to have a better understanding of those afflicted. Women as new and growing victims of the disease face a far greater impact than men. In addition to a feeling of stigmatization common to most HIV-positive people women face several unique problems. They may, for example, experience feelings of extreme isolation, reproductive concerns and fears or guilt about transmitting the virus to their children. Positive women face rejection as marital partner, loss of security and their roles as mothers, daughters, wives or sisters (Buckingam and Rehm, 1987; Chachkes, 1987; Waxler, 1989). In this context, it is important to understand how social workers view women's rights to reproductive freedom and gender equality in sexual and contraceptive decisions. While a few studies have been conducted on college students in India to assess their knowledge and attitudes regarding HIV/AIDS-related issues, there is hardly any empirical data concerning social workers' knowledge, attitudes and concerns regarding HIV/AIDS. It is also not known how adequately social work students in India are prepared to respond to the unique constellation of issues experienced by specific affected groups. AIDS poses a formidable challenge for social workers not simply in terms of what can be done on behalf of clients, but also how to respond professionally. The current study was undertaken to gain a better understanding of social workers' attitudes, knowledge and their level of comfort in working with this patient population and to find out how well they are prepared in social work programmes.

Sample

The sample comprised 385 second-year graduate social work students enrolled in eleven colleges located in four states, two (Maharashtra and Karnataka) being high HIV/AIDS prevalence states and two (Delhi and Haryana) having low to medium incidence of HIV/AIDS cases. The number of schools, their locations and the sample size are described in Table 10.1.

TABLE 10.1 : Sample Description

State	*City*	*# of Colleges*	*Sample Size (N)*
	Mumbai	2	140
Maharashtra	Pune	2	56
	Nagpur	2	60
Karnataka	Bangalore	2	36
Delhi	New Delhi/Delhi	2	60
Haryana	Kurukshetra	1	33
Total =	**6**	**11**	**385**

The four states represented 45% of all graduate social work programmes in the country and were clustered within a geographic proximity that facilitated economical travel given the limited budget and time. In the light of India's great diversity these states were by no means representative of all the social work programmes in the country. However, the four states did provide variations in the sample with respect to religion, culture, sexual mores and exposure to AIDS information. Another consideration also guided the choice of the four states. It was assumed that the schools that were located in the high HIV-prevalence states (Maharashtra, Karnataka) would likely be more sensitive to the AIDS issues than those located in low to medium prevalence states such as Delhi and Haryana. Thus, the cross sampling of the colleges permitted comparison of students in terms of knowledge, attitudes and awareness of the risk. Selection of the second-year students was guided by the following rationale. These students had gone through the bulk of the curriculum and had the opportunity to take electives that could have included content on HIV/AIDS-related issues and ethical dilemmas in working with marginalized clients. Also, they had completed their practicals increasing the possibility that some students might have been in close contact with HIV/AIDS patients.

The sample included more females (59%) than males (41%). Most (84.2%) were unmarried and young with a mean age = 21.2 years. Seven out of ten (70.7%) students identified themselves as Hindus or Sikhs; one out of five students (20.5%) as Christian; 5.2% as Muslims, and 3.4 per cent reported no religious affiliation. Compared to the general population of India, Hindu/Sikhs and Muslims were under represented by almost 18 and six percentage points respectively. Christians, who constitute 2.4 per cent in the overall population, were substantially over represented in the sample that could be attributed to their heavy concentration in Mumbai and Nagpur. Six out of ten (60.1%) students claimed to be either very religious or religious. Overall, the students belonged to middle to upper middle class families with three-fourths of the respondents' fathers being in managerial or professional jobs. Mothers of about 40% of them had obtained graduate or post-graduate degrees.

Procedure

The information was collected anonymously using a pre-tested questionnaire that was personally administered in classroom settings. The questions included a knowledge test and 4 Likert type response scales to assess students' attitudes toward persons with HIV/AIDS, their perception of personal risk and views on gender equality. The instrument also contained questions on demographic characteristics and twenty items to check response consistency. Two professors at Memorial University and one from McGill University who had extensively researched issues related to HIV/AIDS were asked to check the questionnaire for content validity and relevance of the questions.

The heads of the sample colleges were contacted by a letter explaining the purpose of the study and the procedure to be used for collecting information, and inviting them to participate. The letter was followed by a phone call which gave the heads an opportunity to clarify any questions. The response of the heads was highly positive and enthusiastic. In each college the class of the second year students was informed about the study in advance of our meeting and told that the participation was voluntary. As far as could be determined from class instructors the entire class agreed to participate in the survey. In order to promote candid responding, faculty members were politely asked to leave the room during administration and more space was provided between seats to allow privacy. The survey was preceded by an half-hour rapport-building chat which helped create a relaxed, non-threatening atmosphere. To further encourage candid responses and avoid identification of students, the students were instructed to place the answer sheets in an envelop in a corner of the room.

Instrument

Students' knowledge about the transmission, symptomotology, prognosis, and prevention of HIV/AIDS was assessed by a 28 -item test (Cronbach's alpha= .72). A 13-item scale assessed students' attitudes towards persons with HIV/AIDS (alpha = .95). To assess perception of risk of the disease participants responded to a 9-item scale (alpha = .78). Views on gender equality were assessed by a 10-item scale (Cronbach's alpha = .87) and 8 items tested the level of homophobia (Cronbach's alpha = .83). The knowledge and attitude scales, thus, had a high internal consistency among items. The test items utilized in the knowledge and attitude scales occurred most commonly in the pool of items drawn from instruments developed by Dhooper et al. (1987–88), DiClemente et al. (1987), Gray and Saracino (1991), Kelly et al. (1987), National Survey of Adolescent Males (Institute for Survey Research, 1988), Stall and McKusick (1988). As a further measure of reliability of the attitude scales, split-half method was applied by randomly dividing the items into two halves. The correlation of the two subsets ranged from .91 to .95 for the four attitude scales. The test-retest reliability of the measurement scales administered at a three-week interval to the same students in the two colleges in Delhi ranged from .85 to .87 indicating that the instrument was very stable.

Each question in the knowledge scale was answered either true, false or don't know. The "don't know" response option was provided to reduce the guessing factor and was treated as an incorrect answer. The total score for each student was obtained by adding the number of correct answers. The scores ranged from 0 to 28 with a mean score of 21.16 (SD= 3.97). The scores of each student were converted to Z scores which ranged from -5.33 to 1.72. The students were classified into three HIV/AIDS knowledge categories: poor knowledge (Z = less than zero or 75% or less correct answers); good knowledge (Z = 0 to less than 1 or 78% - 85% correct answers), and excellent knowledge (Z =1 to 1.7 or 89% or better correct answers). This is, however, an arbitrary classification reflecting the level of knowledge about HIV/AIDS among these students. The 28-item knowledge inventory contained questions that could be answered from common sense or rudimentary information. However, a few questions regarding etiology of the disease, symtomology and treatment were determined as critical. Knowing these items was highly important for those working with people having the disease. Sixteen such questions were identified. A score of 80% or better on the critical knowledge items was considered satisfactory.

Scores on the attitude sub-scales were computed for each student by assigning a value of 1 through 4 for response options (1=strongly disagree to 4=strongly agree) with higher scores indicating a more positive response. The mean score for each respondent was obtained by summing the four levels of agreement across the items and then dividing by 4. Thus, the minimum possible mean score of an individual was 1 and the maximum was 4. Based on their mean scores the sample students were arbitrarily divided into three equal categories of attitudes: conservative (# 1.99), moderate (2.0 # x # 2.99) and liberal (3.0# x 4.0). One way ANOVA was conducted to determine if there were significant differences in the mean knowledge and attitudes by school, gender, age, marital status and religious affiliation. A Scheffe test was performed to examine pair-wise comparisons between the group means. Chi-square was used to test significance of the difference between proportions. Hierarchical regression analyses were used to locate variables predictive of attitudes toward PWHA, gender equality and perception of risk.

Results

Overall, the students demonstrated a moderate degree of knowledge about HIV/AIDS. Less than one-half (47.5%) had poor knowledge with 75% or less correct answers; three out of ten (31.2%) students were classed as having good knowledge with a score of 78% to 85% correct answers. Only one-fifth (21.3%) had excellent AIDS knowledge having identified 89.3% or more correct answers. In terms of students' knowledge of critical items, only 46% approached the satisfactory level of 80% or better correct answers. Across colleges, the students from Nagpur, Pune (in the state of Maharashtra) and from Haryana were least knowledgeable with 90.4%, 68.3% and 60.6% respectively in the "poor" knowledge category. The students in Bangalore had the fourth lowest scores at 52.8% . The most informed students were from colleges in Delhi with 80% having good to excellent knowledge followed by students in Mumbai with 69.4%. The differences were statistically significant ($X^2(10)=96.527, p< .000$) (see Table 10.2). However, with respect to knowledge of critical items, pair wise comparisons of mean scores shows that while students from Delhi were as knowledgeable as their counterparts in Mumbai, students from both cities showed a higher knowledge compared to the students in all other schools $F(5, 384=18.99, p < .000)$.

Mean knowledge scores significantly differed with respect to gender, marital status and religion. Females obtained somewhat higher mean knowledge scores than males (21.665 vs 20.424, $F(1, 385=9.29, p < .002)$ and married students scored considerably lower than their unmarried counterparts (19.197 vs 21.553, $F(1,383=18.96, p < .000)$. This finding is not surprising considering that the married people generally engage in monogamous relationships with a known sex partner, and thus do not feel the same concern for seeking more information to avoid the risk of HIV infection as do the unmarried people who are not likely to be familiar with the sexual history of their potential sex partners. Among students indicating religious affiliation, Christians obtained significantly higher mean knowledge scores (22.532), compared to either Muslims (21.558) or Hindus/Sikhs (20.677) ($F(2, 384)=7.09$, $p < .001$). However, Scheffe's test revealed that while Christians were as knowledgeable as Hindu/Sikh students, both groups had higher knowledge compared to their Muslim counterparts.

While students' AIDS knowledge was positively related to the educational status of both parents, mothers' educational status seemed to have a stronger impact on the students' degree of knowledge than did the fathers' educational attainment. For example, 63.6% of the students whose fathers had attained master's or better degrees had good to excellent knowledge ($X^2(4) = 25.61$, $p < .000$), whereas 71.7% of the students had good to excellent knowledge whose mothers had the same educational status ($X^2(4) = 34.87$, $p < .000$). Conversely, the level of knowledge dropped considerably when the parents had completed high school or less. These findings suggest that educated mothers have a stronger influence on shaping the information reservoir of their children than do the educated fathers.

Attitudes

Attitude toward People living with HIV/AIDS (PWHA)

In general, the students were moderately empathic toward people living with HIV/AIDS (mean score = 2.18, SD = .864; minimum 0 = 1, maximum 0 = 4). Almost six out of ten students (58.7%) were not supportive in their attitudes having a mean score of # 1.92. Less than 30 per cent (28.6%) held positive attitudes with a mean score of 3.0–4.0. A little over one-tenth (12.7%) were uncertain. The mean differences among colleges were not statistically significant indicating that the students

TABLE 10.2 : Degree of HIV/AIDS Knowledge by Schools

(% Distribution)

Degree of knowledge	*ALL (385)*	*Kurukh-shetra (33) # school =1*	*Delhi (60) # school = 2*	*Mumbai (144) # school =2*	*Nagpur (52) # school 2*	*Pune (60) # school 2*	*Banga-lore (36) # school 2*
Poor [Z score = Less than zero] (75% or less correct ans.)	47.5	60.6	20.2	30.6	90.4	68.3	52.8
Good [Z score = 0 to less than 1] (78%-85% correct ans)	31.2	30.3	38.3	39.6	7.7	28.3	25.0
Excellent [Z score = 1 to 1.72] (89% or more correct ans)	21.3	9.1	41.7		1.9	3.3	22.2

X (10) = 107.96, p < .000 Mean = 21.6, SD = 3.97, Range = 0–28

Note **:** Scheffe's test revealed that there were no significant differences in the mean knowledge scores between the schools in each of the cities. Therefore, the two schools were combined for analysis purpose. Combining schools in each city also served to protect their anonymity.

regardless of the geographic region held a moderately supportive attitude toward HIV/AIDS victims. Females.with 31.8% were slightly more empathic, than males (23.9%) ($X^2(2)$ =10.94, $p < .05$). Students' attitudes toward PWHA were not influenced by gender or marital status, but religious affiliation did make a difference in their attitudes. Christians with 53.9% showed more positive attitudes than either Muslims (37.2%) or Hindus/Sikhs (37.1%) ($X^2(4) = 15.596$, $p < .004$). Parents' educational status had no influence on their attitudes. Note that females, unmarried and Christian students scored higher on mean knowledge than did the male, married and Hindus/ Sikh students. Does accurate information influence attitudes?

As is shown in Table 10.3, knowledge and attitudes are positively related, that is, more knowledgeable students were more empathic toward PWHA and vice versa.

TABLE 10.3 : Students' Knowledge About AIDS and Attitude Toward AIDS Patients

(% Distribution)

		Attitude Toward HIV/AIDS Patients		
Degree of knowledge	*l* (385)	*Conservative* # 1.99	*Moderate* 2.0# x # 2.99	*Liberal* 3.0# x # 4.0
Poor [Z score = Less than zero] (75% or less correct ans.)	46.8	51.8	66.7	27.8
Good [Z score = 0 to less than 1] (78%–85% correct ans)	31.7	30.6	22.9	38.0
Excellent [Z score = 1 to 1.72] (89% or more correct ans)	21.4	17.6	10.4	34.3

X^2 (4) = 28.716, $p < .000$

Based on previous studies it was reasonable to assume that AIDS-related knowledge, sense of competence, adequacy of formal instructions (step 1), contact with HIV/AIDS patients, personal relationship with gay friends, marital status (step 2), religious affiliation, religiousness, mother's education and father's education (step 3), would predict attitude toward PWHA (Melkote and Goswami., 2000; Selvan et al., 2001; Weiner and Siegel, 1990). Linear regression analysis using the stepwise method was employed to locate the predictors. The analysis indicated that three independent predictors emerged as statistically significant. These are listed in order of their relative strength of influence on attitude toward PWHA:

'personal relationships with gay/lesbian friends' ($ = .48, p < .000),'sense of competence'($ =-.45, p < .000), and 'actual contact with AIDS patients' ($ =.15, p < .000). ® square = .46; Adjusted R square = .44) These variables together explain 46% of the variance in attitude toward PWHA.

Self-Perception of Risk

In general, the students showed a lack of serious concern for contracting the disease. (mean score=2.143, SD=.6335; min.0 =1 max.0 =4)). Close to one-half (48.3%) were determined to have low perception of risk with a mean of # 1.99. A little over one-third (36.6%) had a moderate concern (mean 2.0 # 2.99). Less than one in ten (15.1%) expressed a high fear of the contagion (3.0 # 4.0). Put differently, the students were almost divided between those having low concern (48.3%) and those with moderate to high awareness of the risk (51.7%). The colleges did not significantly differ from each other on the level of concern for the disease (F(5,384), .594, p >.05). Paradoxically, almost one half (45% to 50%) of all the students from the state of Maharashtra, the high HIV prevalence area, had a low concern about contracting the AIDS virus. This finding is in agreement with the global survey commissioned by BBC. The survey noted that in spite of a real risk of major AIDS disaster, only one-third of the respondents in India thought that HIV/AIDS was their main concern (*BBC News* (World edition), 16 November 2003).

Gender and marital status did not make any difference in the level of awareness of the risk of AIDS infection. However, religion did influence the degree of awareness, with Christians being the most concerned (59.5%) and Muslims the least concerned (62.8%) ($X^2(4)$=15.981, p < . 003). The Hindu/Sikh students were second to Christian students with more than one half (51.7%) being aware of the risk. AIDS knowledge was significantly related to perception of personal risk, that is those who were more knowledgeable were also more concerned about contracting the AIDS virus (see Table 10.4).

TABLE 10.4 : Students' Knowledge About AIDS and Perception of Risk

(% Distribution)

Degree of Knowledge	*Perception of Risk* ALL (385)	*Low Awareness # 1.99*	*Moderate Awareness 2.0# X # 2.99*	*High Awareness 3.0# x # 4.0*
Poor [Z score = Less than zero] (75% or less correct ans.)	47.5	54.6	49.5	24.1
Good [Z score = 0 to less than 1] (78%–85% correct ans)	31.2	29.1	31.7	34.5
Excellent [Z score = 1 to 1.72] (89% or more correct ans)	21.3	16.3	18.8	41.4

X^2 (4) = 21.895, p < .000

A hierarchical multiple regression model was used to determine the study assumption that the students' perceived risk for the disease was influenced by the following variables: AIDS-related knowledge, sense of competence, adequacy of instructions in the MSW program, mother's education, father's education (step 1); contact with HIV/AIDS patients, woman's control over contraceptive decision, acceptability for carrying condoms by women, personal relationships with gay friends (step 2); gender, religious affiliation, religiousness and marital status (step 3). The analysis in step 1 revealed that only 'sense of competence' emerged as a significant predictor (∃ = .-450, p < .000). In step 2 'personal relationships with gay friends' was the most powerful predictor (∃ = .42, p .< .000), followed by 'actual contact with AIDS patients' (∃ = .112, p < .009). The correlation between woman's control over contraceptive decision and individual's perceived risk of the disease was statistically significant, but relatively weak (∃ = .083, p < .05). These variables combined accounted for 39% of the variance (R square = .39; Adjusted R square = .37).

Gender Equality

Overall, the students had a moderate to high acceptance of gender equality at 90.6 per cent (mean score=2.784, SD=.6006; min 0= 1, max 0 =4.). Their robust support for gender equality could be attributed to the humanitarian values and social work philosophy that is rooted in egalitarian principles and social justice which enable them to have a better understanding of women as an oppressed class. Across colleges, the students from Pune and Nagpur had the lowest mean equality acceptance scores at 2.514 and 2.378 respectively. The highest mean scores were obtained by students from Mumbai (2.981) and Delhi (2.962). The students from Bangalore and Haryana were the third and the fourth highest with a mean score of 2.898 and 2.606 respectively, slightly below the Mumbai and Delhi students. The differences in the mean scores were statistically significant [(F,5, 384), 14.297, $p < .000$)]. Chi-square distribution confirms the findings. That is, the highest proportion of students from Mumbai (57.6%) and Delhi (53.4%)were in the "high acceptance" of gender equality category followed by Bangalore (47.2%). The students from Pune and Nagpur were in the lowest proportion with 20% and 13.5% in the same category ($X^2(10) = 53.723$, $p < .000$).

Females were significantly more supportive of gender equality than were males (59.5% vs 15.8%) ($X^2(2) = 74.968$, $p < .000$). Married students were far less supportive compared to unmarried students (24.6% vs 45.0%), ($X^2(2) = 9.423$, $p < .009$). Religious preference significantly affected the students' attitude toward gender equality. Christians at 57% were far more accepting of gender equality than were either Muslims or Hindus/Sikhs who accounted for 39.5% and 37.3% respectively ($X^2(4) = 12.822$, $p < .012$). AIDS knowledge and acceptance of gender equality were positively related, that is more knowledgeable students were more likely to accept gender equality and vice versa (see Table 10.5).

Support for gender equality was assumed to be associated with overall AIDS related knowledge, sense of competence, adequacy of instructions in the MSW programme, father's education, mother's education, gender (step 1), sexual assertiveness, acceptability for carrying condoms by women, equality of sexual freedom, rejection of virginity norms, number of boys/girls dated (step 2), religious affiliation, religiousness, marital status (step 3). Hierarchical (step-wise) multiple regression analyses were conducted to identify which of these variables explained students' support for gender equality. Being female was the most powerful significant predictor (∃ =.-42, $p < .000$). AIDS knowledge (∃ = .24, $p < .02$) and mother's education (∃ = .11, p .< .04) had significant, but weak influence on students' support for gender equality. Furthermore, sexual assertiveness was most influential (∃ = .37, $p < .000$) followed by equality of sexual freedom (∃ = .20, $p < .000$), acceptability of carrying condoms by women (B = .19, $p < .000$), rejection of virginity norms (∃ = .08, $p < .04$). Being Christian emerged as a significant but weak predictor (∃ = .09, p < . 006). The overall R square value (.70) indicated that eight variables accounted for 70% of the variance in the dependent variable. Adjusted R square value was 68.

Attitude towards homosexuality

The students were, generally, opposed to homosexual acts with more than one half (55.5%) being strongly opposed. One-third (34.2%) were moderately supportive. Only one in ten students (10.4%) thought homosexuality was acceptable. Across colleges, the mean scores ranged from 1.951 (Haryana) to 2.0215 (Mumbai) with an overall mean score of 2.0165 (SD= .6002). (The higher mean signifies stronger acceptance of homosexuality). The difference in the mean scores were not significant. More females than males found homosexual acts acceptable ($X^2(2) = 6.901$, $p < .03$). Married students were less likely to approve of homosexuality than were unmarried students ($X^2(2) = 5.775$, $p < .05$). Religion or religiousness did not significantly affect the students' attitude toward homosexual acts. These findings are in accord with previous studies which reported that social workers, generally, felt more negatively about homosexuality since the emergence of AIDS (DeCrescenzo, 1983; Wiener and Siegel, 1990; Wisniewski and Toomey, 1987).

TABLE 10.5 : Students' Knowledge About AIDS and Gender Equality

(% Distribution)

Degree of knowledge	***ALL (385)***	*Gender Equality* Low Acceptance # 1.99	*Moderate Acceptance 2.0# x # 2.99*	*High Acceptance 3.0# x # 4.0*
Poor [Z score = Less than Zero} (75% or less correct ans.)	47.5	58.3	63.5	26.3
Good [Z score = 0 to less than 1] (78%–85% correct ans.)	31.2	25.0	22.2	43.1
Excellent [Z score = 1 to 1.72 (89% or more correct ans.)	21.3	16.7	14.3	30.6

X^2 (4) = 50.150, p < .000

Instructions in knowledge and skills

The students were asked if the school provided them with instructions on HIV/AIDS and counseling skills and how adequate these instructions were. More than one-half (55.3%) received either "absolutely no" instructions on the subject or the instructions were "somewhat" adequate. Four out of ten students (44.7%) described their instructions "adequate" or "very adequate" and reported the total class time spent was less than six hours. Across colleges, the percentages of students who thought the instructions were "adequate" or "very adequate" varied in range between 42% to 50%. In another question students' sense of competence and preparedness was determined by their agreement or disagreement (on a four-point scale) with the statement: "I believe I'm adequately prepared with knowledge and skills in my social work education to work with clients with HIV/AIDS infection."

Three-fourth (76.1%) of the students disagreed with the statement implying their lack of competence. Interestingly, the sense of competence was the lowest among students from Delhi (15%) and Mumbai (20.8%), the schools with the highest knowledge scores. What appears from these findings is that mere factual instructions do not necessarily engender a sense of competence and preparedness and perhaps there are a host of mediating and contextual factors that play a greater role in achieving the impact of accurate information on the sense of competence.

Discussion

The study findings reveal that overall the students had a moderate degree of knowledge about HIV transmission, prevention and its treatment. Only one-fifth were able to identify 86% or more correct answers. Further, less than one-half (46%) of all students were determined to have satisfactory knowledge of the critical items in the knowledge inventory. The finding of great concern is that students from colleges particularly in the high HIV prevalence regions (i.e. Nagpur, Pune) did poorly on the AIDS knowledge scores. As well, the students from the colleges in the high HIV prevalence areas such as Maharashtra and Karnataka were not all that concerned about the risk of the contagion. One would, normally, expect a high level of concern among these students given their proximity to the epicentre. Of course, the students from colleges in Mumbai did better on the AIDS knowledge. However, they did not do as well as one would expect in view of the fact that Mumbai received massive and intensive exposure to educational and awareness campaigns since the first cases of HIV positive were detected more than a decade ago.

Compared to the level of knowledge of the sample students, the social work students in most American surveys had much higher scores having identified 80 to 90 per cent of the correct answers on similar questions (see, for example, Geringer et al., 1993; Gray and Saracino, 1991; Owens, 1995; Waxler, 1980; Wiener and Siegel, 1990). It is possible that the rapid growth of the AIDS pandemic has not prompted new interest and awareness in the social work community. It is disturbing to note that three-fourth of the sample students admitted to their lack of competence and adequate professional preparation to deal with the unique problems that the HIV positive clients and their families present. This finding is consistent with a general survey of social work students in the US that reported their respondents were not sure if they were cognitively and affectively prepared to deal with AIDS-related issues (Diaz and Kelly, 1991; Gillman, 1991; Owens, 1995; Peterson, 1991; Silberman, 1991; Waxler, 1989; Wiener and Siegel, 1990). This finding is not surprising since only one-quarter (26.8%) of them received formal instructions in their graduate programmes, while magazines were the primary source of information for almost four out of ten (38.1.%) students. The moderate level of knowledge and low anxiety for the disease among our participants is supported by studies on college students in India (Amalraj et al., 1995; Bharat, 1996; Kumar et al., 1997). The findings of this study and those of others point out to a distressing fact that the educational and awareness campaigns of government and non-government agencies (e.g., NGOs) have not impacted on a large segments of young people, the new vulnerable group. This makes sense when one considers that India's National AIDS Control Organization's (NACO) awareness campaigns so far has been exclusively focusing on the high risk groups identified as commercial sex workers, truck drivers and IV drug users. Those outside these target groups, the young women and men in the mainstream of the population, were not considered a priority. This observation is supported by NACO's behavioural survey which revealed that awareness levels, knowledge of HIV transmission and perceived risk to self were low among the general population, especially among women (NACO, 2001).

Although the study observed that AIDS-related knowledge influences perception of risk, the Social Influence Theory advanced by Fisher (1988) posits that the influence of knowledge attenuates in the presence of certain socio-environmental factors such as behavioural norms and values.

Norms and beliefs about how their peers and the role models in movies and the television sitcoms generate a normative behaviour standard to which individuals aspire and conform to, risky or not. Some psychologists, however, prefer to explain perception of risk under the cognitively and rationally based perception processes as in the Health Belief Model (Becker, 1974). According to them, an individual appraises risk either cognitively or emotionally. For example, an individual may cognitively comprehend risk of the disease, yet be unconcerned emotionally. In other words, there is a real distinction between being 'worried' about the disease, and actually believing that the individual might contract that disease. Eagly (1992) argues that unless individuals are motivated to do otherwise, information is processed at a superficial level. Markova et al. (1995) posit that what is and what is not considered risky is also determined by the manner in which individuals attribute blame for the disease. The perception in the public's mind still persists that AIDS is a disease confined to deviant groups, i.e., prostitutes, gays, IV drug users, promiscuous heterosexuals. This belief serves the purpose of reducing personal anxiety over risk of infection as the individual does not identify herself/himself with such deviant groups. This theoretical framework is very instructive for social work educators. They should make sure that social workers gain in-depth knowledge specific to AIDS and STI (sexually transmitted infections), but, more importantly, the instruction should address students' emotion, sentiments and personal prejudices concerning HIV+/AIDS patients.

In the current study, participants showed a low level of comfort in working with HIV/AIDS patients in spite of having knowledge of the disease. This is also confirmed by the students' response to the individual attitudinal items. Close to one-half (47.2%) disagreed with the statement: "I wouldn't mind if one of my classmates had AIDS and continued to attend classes". More than four out of ten (45.2%) would hesitate to work with clients having AIDS. Four out of ten students blamed AIDS victims for their disease. This finding is congruent with most of the American investigations

(Bulter, 1990; Owens, 1992; Riley and Greene, 1993; Royse and Birge, 1987; Rubin et al., 1996; Silberman, 1991; Wexler, 1989; Wiener and Siegel, 1990). These studies as well as the present study demonstrate that accurate knowledge is necessary, but not a sufficient condition to influence attitude toward HIV/ AIDS patients. Students may have intellectually accepted persons with AIDS, believing they are free of biases or prejudices. Clearly, teaching strategies should incorporate an affective module that allows students to freely sift through values regarding HIV/AIDS infected people and help them internalize these beliefs. The framework entitled "Identifying the isms" developed by Latting (1990) can be used to enable students to willingly admit having biases and work through them by way of group discussion. Repeated exposure to information coupled with discussion sessions have proven more effective in increasing students' comfort level than short minimal educational programmes (e.g., a lecture) (Barr et al., 1992; Lipson and Brown, 1991; Rotheram-Bonus et al., 1998; Slomin-Nevo et al., 1991; Weisse et al., 1995). Consistent with previous investigations, the regression analysis failed to support AIDS-related knowledge alone as a significant predictor. But it identified personal relationships with gay friends, sense of competence and actual contact with AIDS patients as strong predictors of attitude toward PWHA. Admittedly, variable 'personal relationships with gay/lesbian friends' is non-manipulable. What is feasible is that an educational strategy can be designed so that it encourages students to do projects or field placements which can bring them in direct contact with HIV-positive persons and AIDS victims. This approach has demonstrated that students move beyond the intellectual level and develop better understanding, greater sensitivity and empathy toward the patients (Bliwise, 1991; Miller & Dane, 1990; Scollary et al., 1992). The current study reveals that by and large the students had negative attitude toward homosexuality and males were more prejudicial than females. The training programme must include in-depth discussion of homosexuality and an opportunity for students, and in particular the male students, to explore their prejudices. Inviting guest lecturers from the gay/lesbian community has proved quite helpful in removing stereotypical views about homosexuals.

The high prevalence of HIV infection among commercial sex workers is a major challenge to health care providers. Given the unequal power relations sex workers are unable or unwilling to insist on the use of condoms by their male clients. According to a survey conducted in a red light area in Kolkata, called Sonagachi, only 1.5% of the clients regularly used condoms (Nath, 2000). In addition, government laws criminalize commercial sex work and its premises which subject sex workers to harassment and police brutality. Under the programme of targeted intervention NACO launched educational and awareness campaigns along with free condom distribution in several red light areas, but these initiatives have had limited success in generating safe sexual practices among sex workers. The main obstacles seem to be the absence of measures such as providing legitimacy to the trade, rescue and rehabilitation opportunities, care and support for those who were infected with HIV/AIDS/STDs, and, above all, a sense of personal security. It would be inconceivable to expect sex workers to have motivation to translate their knowledge into safe sex behaviour and to feel concerned about the safety of personal health in the face of constant fear of eviction and detention (Amin, 2004). More importantly, these women lack an organization with collective power to negotiate with male clients so that if one denies sex to a client who resists using condoms, another would not barter for a higher price. Social workers can apply their advocacy skills in order to help female sex workers gain basic human rights and protection from arbitrary harassment and abuse. Through their skills in group dynamics and community organization social workers can play a vital role in helping them organize into a collective body which can enhance their power of negotiation with clients and owners of brothels. One such shining example is the sex workers of Sonagachi in Kolkata. Through their collectivism they have been highly effective in practising safer sex. This has significantly decreased the incidence of HIV and improved the sex workers' overall health (Nath, 2000).

Some instructors might avoid giving instructions on AIDS because of their discomfort with the subject of sex which plays a key role in the understanding of the transmission of HIV virus, reproductive tracts infections and HIV-risk reduction interventions. As far as can be determined there are no formal instructions on human sexuality in schools and universities in India and the stigma associated with sex has forced youth to depend on informal channels. In a study of 887 students from two major universities in Delhi, India this author found that more than eight out of ten students received information about sex from "the street", i.e., friends or sex manuals (Sachdev, 1997, 1998). The country is still caught up in a bitter debate whether there should be sex education in schools and colleges. Paradoxically, there is a taboo on the discussion of sex in Indian society, yet young people live in a highly sexually charged environment fulled largely by explicit portrayal of sexual intimacy, exotic and sexually suggestive dances, and sensuous rap songs and lyrics.

Interestingly, while the condom is, presently, the only viable means of preventing HIV transmission, the policy of the government of India prohibits explicit references to condoms in schools and colleges or their display on billboards or in the mass media (*The Financial Times,* 21 December 2003). Even the government-sponsored educational and awareness campaigns squeamishly mention the word "sex" *(New York Times,* 30 November 2003). The governor of Bihar would not endorse any reference to condoms in educational campaigns, because according to him condoms encourage immoral sex in the society (*Times News Network,* 16 December 2003). There is an oddity in that we are dealing with the HIV/AIDS epidemic and its prevention through the use of condoms which are inevitably linked with the discussion of sex. A well-structured AIDS education should integrate information on sexual anatomy and its functioning, and sex-related issues such as sexual arousal, desires and mutual masturbation with the content on AIDS. It should focus on the students' own feelings and attitudes regarding variant sexual behaviours. Techniques such as de-sensitization, role plays and rehearsals are quite effective in making the students aware of their own sexual values, inhibitions, guilt feelings and resolving them through discussions, feedback from participants and self-exploration. The goal of sex education is to enable students to foster interaction with HIV/AIDS clients and their partners without prejudices and hang-ups.

While HIV/AIDS is a health issue, the epidemic is a gender issue. Over 80% of HIV infections are transmitted through sexual relations between women and men. Epidemiologists agree that HIV-positive young women are expected to outnumber their seropositive male peers by as much as six times because of their physiological susceptibility and unequal power relation vis-á-vis men (UNIFEM, 2003; UNFPA, 2002). This ominous trend, therefore, supports the strategic need to address gender roles and power dynamics between women and men and, their impact on sexual relations and decision-making. This strategy is crucial for effective prevention. Because of early socialization, women learn to be submissive and conformist to their husbands/boy friends' preferences. The problem of unequal power relationships and lack of assertiveness is highlighted even by well-educated upper middle to upper class women in this study. Almost 50 per cent (47.1%) admitted that they would be afraid of offending their husbands if they asked them to use condoms despite their knowledge that they had been engaging in risky sexual behaviours. The female condom is one device that can offer women control over contraceptive and sexual decisions. However, this method is either not available or is very expensive for middle and lower economic class women which leaves the only preventive device available for them is the male condom. The male condom puts the onus on the male for its use. Moreover, not only do men find condoms inconvenient, they also think that contraception is the female's responsibility (Freeman et al., 1980; Gough, 1979; Sachdev, 1993). In this study, only a little more than one third (36.7%) of male students disagreed with the statement: " It's a woman's responsibility to take control of contraception if she wants to protect herself against the AIDS virus."

Trained students should have conviction in and commitment to women's rights to express their sexual and assertiveness needs as men do. A surprising and unsettling finding of the study was that male social work students had great reservations in accepting equality among genders. Since many of the male graduates are going to work with female clients, the educators in social work should ascertain that students develop a more positive and supportive attitude toward gender equality, a sine qua non for gaining trust of their female clients. Such an attitude is imperative irrespective of their level of practice (direct practice, community development, policy or administration) since each area of practice is impacted by women's issues.

Women's empowerment is the only HIV vaccine available today. Women's empowerment includes extending to them all fundamental social, economic and political rights which are guaranteed under legislation in India. However, at the individual level, women are either unwilling or unable to exercise these rights because of socio-cultural constraints, traditions, family values and deeply rooted practices that apply to women and men differently. This increases women's vulnerability to HIV infection. Results from the regression analysis reveal that sexual assertiveness of females and equality of sexual freedom are the most influential variables that impact on gender equality. Social workers should be trained to design women-specific initiatives that facilitate the empowerment process whereby women challenge the effects of gender-based disadvantages and learn self-regulative skills such as communication on sexuality and reproductive health. These skills would enable women to negotiate safer sex and be assertive to refuse coitus, if necessary. An educational and awareness programme aimed at behaviour change can hardly succeed unless men are actively involved and are encouraged to understand that women are human beings who have feelings and specific needs. In men-only groups social workers can create opportunities for openly discussing concerns, pressures, emotions in relation to males engaging in behaviours that place them and their female partners at risk of HIV/AIDS. The active participation of specialized women's groups as well as people living with HIV/AIDS at all levels of programming has proved very effective in promoting empowerment and autonomy of girls and women (International Conference of South Asian Parliamentarians, New Delhi, 1–2 August 2003). While changing unequal gender relationships is a long-term process and cannot be achieved through awareness programs alone, gender sensitive HIV/AIDS prevention measures do play a critical role in promoting equitable norms (Amin, 2004).

There is yet no cure for HIV/AIDS; a preventive vaccine has eluded scientists and anti-retroviral drugs, which do not cure AIDS but enhance the quality of life of the patients, are too expensive for most of the people in India. In view of this, the experts recommend that prevention through behaviour change seems to be the best and most feasible approach to reverse the epidemic (Selvan et al., 2001; Yang, 2003; UNFPA, 2001). This approach is based on the research findings that standard HIV/AIDS education and changes in attitudes may be necessary, but are not sufficient conditions for reducing HIV/AIDS risk behaviour (Meskote and Goswami, 2000; Shveller and Pietersma, 2002; Scalway, 2003:20; Walter et al., 1992). The government strategy advocates the ABC approach, that is, abstinence (A) be faithful to one's partner (B) and use condom (C), if the adherence to the first two behavioural changes are not feasible. There are so far no empirical data that suggest whether this intervention strategy has proven effective in reducing HIV risk behaviours. However, a few controlled studies conducted in North America have reported behavioural outcomes indicative of sustained HIV/AIDS risk reduction behaviour change among young people (Bryan et al., 1996; Fisher et al, 1996; Jermott et al., 1999; Lawrence et al., 1995; 1996; 1999; Rotheram-Bonus et al., 1998). They demonstrated that the groups which received education coupled with social skills training based on cognitive behavioural principles engaged in considerably less unprotected sex, developed more favourable attitudes toward condom use, greater sexual communication and deferred the onset of sexual activity to a greater extent than youths who received HIV/AIDS information only. The behavioural principles included correct condom use, sexual assertiveness to be able to refuse sexual initiation or to resist coercion, positive reactions to condoms, communication with a sex partner on the importance of safer sex, sexual values, risk recognition, and AIDS prevention motivation.

Interestingly, most of the studies of effective intervention shared key common elements, e.g., social learning and cognitive behaviour theories as their conceptual frameworks, equal emphasis on abstinence and lowering risk behaviour. Instructional techniques included sexual assertion role play, peer educators and simulated exercises, rehearsal, modelling and communication skills. A "well-rounded" social worker equipped with skills in evaluation procedures can use the conceptual framework and behavioural skills identified by these studies as guidelines for evaluating the behavioural outcomes in their clients as a consequence of their prevention interventions. The use of evaluation is consistent with the social workers' responsibility to assess whether their interventions to prevent HIV risk behaviour has yielded desired outcomes and thus to demonstrate their accountability to the funding agency. There is a growing expectation on the part of governmental agencies that HIV prevention interventions mirror tangible evidence that ultimately transmission of HIV has slowed down or halted. The social worker who understands and employs evaluation to validate change is viewed as demonstrating concern for his /her clients (Rubin and Babbie, 2001:10). Making a difference in clients' lives is the hallmark of good practice and is compatible with professional ethics.

Schools of Social Work might also provide training opportunities for the faculty members to update their knowledge of AIDS-related and sexual issues, to examine their biases as well as learn innovative training strategies. Students' ability to internalize knowledge greatly depends upon the instructor's level of comfort with the subject, and his/her own fears and prejudices.

Teaching content on AIDS can be achieved in a variety of ways. The content can be integrated into the core courses or offered as elective or selective topic courses. The Canadian Association of Schools of Social Workers (CASSW) developed a curriculum guide on HIV / AIDS education for social workers. Its main recommendations are that the following content areas must form the base of AIDS education: *AIDS-specific facts* (e.g., etiology, transmission, prevention); *politics of AIDS*; *assessment; intervention* (e.g., behaviour change, sexual assertiveness, support, peer educators); *action* (e.g., advocacy); *specialized counselling* to assist patients and their significant others to cope with the disease and treatment (e.g., pre and post-testing, spirituality, death and (bereavement); *specialized issues* (e.g., human sexuality, homophobia, sexism), *values clarification, ethics, confidentiality, discrimination, gender issues, civil rights*. Four considerations must be raised here: First, curriculum content must involve an interplay of knowledge, attitudes, skills and values in every discussion of AIDS. Second, as much as possible the community, especially PWHA, should be involved in teaching and learning. Third, field placement opportunities need to be provided to students who wish to develop further their interest in AIDS. Fourth, the development and implementation of special topic course(s) would offer an opportunity to those students who wish to concentrate in this area (CASSW, 1990). Preliminary evidence suggests that regardless of format of the curriculum, quality of a programme that emphasizes in-depth exploration of issues, rather than its duration, is more likely to produce measurable improvement in appropriate attitudes, knowledge and professional skills (Lipson and Brown, 1991; Scollay et al.,1992).

Limitations

Any attempts at generalization from the findings of this study should be mindful of the convenience sample used in the study. India is diverse in contextual, socio-cultural factors, traditions and values. States also differ with respect to the level of exposure to HIV education and awareness campaigns and risk reduction programs. It is quite likely that because of these factors social work students in other states could exhibit marked differences from the students in this study in terms of HIV prevention knowledge, attitudes, the level of anxiety about the disease and the level of preparedness. It is recognized that conducting research on a country-wide basis might be prohibitive because of the financial cost. Alternatively, future investigators might select colleges of social work from different regions and the results from these studies could be compared with the findings of this study. The future research should focus on the psycho-social and cultural barriers Indian women face in exercising their equal rights and control over contraception and sexual matters. Mail questionnaires do not have the same advantages as do the personally administered questionnaires. The latter ensures a much higher response rate and better quality data (Bailey,1987; Neuman, 2000; Rubin and Babbie, 2001). The self-administered questionnaire employed in this study contained items that were of intimate personal nature and the responses obtained through self-report measures might have been under-reported or exaggerated because of the social desirability effect. However, several cross-check questions built into the instrument indicated very minimal inconsistencies. Also, we believe that several measures such as a creation of psychologically safe environment, good rapport, safeguard against unwanted intrusion or distractions from classmates, assurance of confidentiality and anonymity and emphasis on the importance of truthful responses could have sharply reduced the possibility of response bias.

Limited time and money did not allow travel to many states to include more colleges in the sample. However, to obtain variability in the experience of these students the colleges selected were in the states that contrasted widely with each other. Furthermore, the findings of this study compare well with those reported by investigations conducted on college students and surveys carried out by national and international agencies in India.

Given the limitations, this preliminary study does suggest several salient avenues for enhancing social workers' capacity to respond to the AIDS pandemic. First, it underscores the need for more in-depth and comprehensive presentation of HIV/AIDS-specific knowledge as well as an affective exploration of attitudes. Second, acceptance of and commitment to gender equality, especially among male students should be of high priority when disseminating educational content. Several experts agree that gender inequalities play a critical role in fuelling the epidemic and need to be addressed in programmes focused on women, including sex workers (Annan, 2001; Amin, 2004). Third, training strategies must focus on social skills based on learning and cognitive behavioural theory to implement behaviour change. The HIV epidemic dynamic is not simply viewed in terms of treatment options, prevention strategies, but as sexual behaviour which is widely diverse and deeply embedded in individual desires, social and cultural relationships and economic processes. Thus, behaviour change is the only remedy to halt the rapid growth of the pandemic. Using gender and culture-sensitive HIV risk-reduction intervention based on the knowledge of social cognitive theory (Bandura, 1986, 1994), the theory of reasoned action (Ajzen and Fishbein, 1980; Fishbein and Ajzen, 1975) and the theory of planned behaviour (Ajzen, 1991; Madden et al., 1992) social workers can play a vital role in reducing risky sexual behaviours. Several investigators who proposed and applied these theories have demonstrated sustained reduction in risky sexual behaviours, increase in self-efficacy and the efficacy of condoms, and in awareness about the risk from the disease among adolescent population (See for example, Jermmott et al., 1999). Finally, the results of this study highlight the need for assessment of the HIV/AIDS curricula to gauge their effectiveness.

Acknowledgment

The author extends deepest gratitude to the heads of all participating colleges of social work for their excellent cooperation and support in collecting information for the study. Appreciations are extended to Professor Henry Schulz and Mr. Gerry White for their valuable assistance in data analysis. Thanks with gratitude to Professor Norm Garlie for his immensely helpful editorial comments. Thanks to Shastri Indo–Canadian Institute for providing funding support for the project.

REFERENCES

Abraham, L. (2001). Understanding youth sexuality. *The Indian Journal of Social Work,* 62(2) (April): 233–248.

Aggrawal, O., Sharma, A.K. and Chabra, P. (2000). "Study in Sexuality of Medical College Students in India." *Journal of Adolescent Health*: 26, 226–229.

Ajzen, I. (1991). *The theory of planned behavior. Organizational behavior and human decision processes,* 50: 179–211.

Ajzen, I. and Fishbein, M. (1980). *Understanding attitudes and predicting social behavior.* Englewood Cliffs: NJ: Prentice Hall.

Amalraj, E.R., Chandrasekaran, N., Solomon, S. and Sambandam, R.P. (1995). First year medical students' AIDS knowledge and attitude, *Indian Journal of Community Medicine,* 20(1-4): 243–246.

Ambati, B.K., Ambati, J. and Rao, A.M. (1997). Dynamics of knowledge and attitudes about AIDS among the educated in Southern India. *AIDS Care,* 9(3): 319–330.

Amin, A. (2004, January). *Risk, Morality, and Blame: A Critical Analysis of Government and U.S. Donor Responses to HIV Infection Among Sex Workers in India.* Takoma Park: MD, Center for Health and Gender Equity.

Anderson, J.L., Kann, D., Holtrzmann, S., Arday, B., Trumen, S. and Kolbe, L. (1990). HIV/AIDS knowledge and sexual behavior among high school students. *Family Planning Perspectives,* 22(6): 252-5.

Annan, K. (2001). *Declaration of Commitment on HIV/AIDS.* The United Nations General Assembly Special Session on HIV/AIDS (UNGASS) A Report. p.88.

Awasthi, S., Nichter, M. and Pande, V.K. (2000). Developing an interactive STD-prevention program for youth: Lessons from a North Indian Slum. *Studies in Family Planning* 31(2): 138–50.

Bailey, K.D. (1987). *Methods of Social Research, 3rd ed.* Toronto: Ontano Free Press.

Bandura, A. (1994). Social cognitive theory and exercise of control over HIV infection. In R. DiClemente & J. Peterson (eds.) *Preventing AIDS: Theories and methods of behavioral interventions* (pp. 25–60): New York: Plenum Press.

Bandura, A. (1986). *Social foundations of thought and action: A social cognitive theory*. Englewood Cliffs, NJ: Prentice-Hall.

Barr, J., Waring and Washaw, L. (1992). Knowledge and attitudes about AIDS among corporate and public service employees. *American Journal of Public Health,* 82(2), 225–8.

Becker, M. (1974). The health belief model and personal health behavior. *Health Education Monograph,* 2, 326–473.

Bharat, S. (1996). *Facing the challenge: household responses to HIV/AIDS in Mumbai, India.* Mumbai: Tata Institute of Social Sciences.

Bourdier, F. (ed.) (1998). *Of Research and Action.* Pondicherry, India: The French Institute of Pondicherry.

Boyer, C.B., Shafer, M. and Tschann, J.M. (1997). Evaluation of a knowledge and behavioral skills building intervention to prevent STDs and HIV infection in high school students. *Adolescence,* 32(125): 25–42.

Bryan, A.D., Aiken, L.S. and West, S.G. (1996). Increasing condom use Evaluation of a theory-based intervention to prevent sexually transmitted diseases in young women. *Health Psyhology,* 15(5): 371–82.

Buckingham, S.L. and Rehm, S.J. (1987). AIDS and women at risk. *Health and Social Work,* 12: 5–11.

Bulter, A.C. (1990). Winter. A reevaluation of social work students' career interests. *Journal of Social Work Education* 1 : 45–56.

Canadian Association of Schools of Social Work. (1990). *HIV/AIDS and Social Work Education: A Curriculum Guide.* Ottawa: Canadian Association of Schools of Social Work.

Chachkes, E. (1987). Women and children with AIDS. In C.G. Leukefeld and M. Fimbres (eds). *Responding to AIDS: Psychosocial Initiatives.* NASW: Silver Spring, MD (p. 5, 64).

Collumbien, M., Das, B. and Campbell, M.R. (2001). Why are condoms used, and how many are needed? Estimates from Orissa, India. *International Family Planning Perspectives* 27(4):171–77.

DeCrescenzo, T. (1983). Homophobia: A study of the attitudes of mental health professional toward homosexuality. *Journal of Social Work and Homosexuality* 2(2-3): 115–36.

Dhooper, S., Royse, D. and Tran.T. (1987–88). Social work practitioners' attitudes toward AIDS victims. *Journal of Applied Social Services,* 12(1): 108–23.

Diaz, Y. and Kelly, J. (1991). AIDS-related training in American schools of social work, *Social Work,* 36: 38–42.

Diaz, Y. and Kelly, J. (1991b). AIDS related training in U.S. schools of social work, *Social Work,* 36(1): 38–42.

DiClemente, R., Zoran, J. and Temoshok. (1987). The association of gender, ethnicity, and length of residence in the bay area of adolescents' knowledge and attitudes about acquired immune deficiency syndrome. *Journal of Applied Social Psychology,* 17: 216–30.

DiClemente, R J. and Wingood, G. (1995). A randomized controlled trial of an HIV sexual risk-reduction intervention for young African-American women. *Journal of American Medical Association,* 274(16): 1271–76.

Dube, S. (2000). *Sex, Lies, and AIDS.* New Delhi: Harper Collins Publishers India.

Eagly, A.H. (1992). Uneven progress: Social psychology and the study of attitudes, *Journal of Personality and Social Psychology,* 62: 693–710.

Fishbein, M. and Ajzen, I. (1975). Belief, attitude, intention an behavior. Boston: Addison-Wesley.

Fisher, J.D. (1988). Possible effects of reference group-based social influence on AIDS-risk behavior and AIDS prevention, *American Psychology,* 43: 914–20.

Freeman, E. et al. (1980). Adolescent contractive use: Comparison of male and female attitudes and information. *American Journal of Public Health,* 70(8): 790–797.

Gagakhedkar, R.R., Bentley, D., Gadkari, M. and Shepherd, B. (1997). *Spread of HIV Infection in Married Monogamous Women in India.* Journal of the American Medical Association, 278(23): 2090–2092.

Geringer, W., Marks, S., Allen, W., and Armstrong, K. (1993). Knowledge, attitudes and behavior related to condom use and STDs in a high risk population, *Journal of Sex Research* 30(1): 75–83.

Gillman, R. (1991). From resistence to rewards: Social workers' experiences and attitudes toward AIDS, *Families in Society,* 72(10): 593–601.

Gough, H. (1979). Some factors related to men's stated unwillingness to use a male contraceptive pill. *Journal of Sex Research* 15(1): 27–37.

Gray, L. and Saracino, M. (1991). AIDS on campus: A preliminary study of college student' knowledge and behavior. *Journal of Counseling and Development,* 68: 1990202. Gray, L., and Sarcino, M. (1991b). College students' attitudes, beliefs, and behaviors about AIDS:Implications for family life educators, *Family Relations* 40 (July): 258–63.

Ismail, S. et al. (1995). Knowledge, attitudes and practice on high risk factors pertaining to HIV/AIDS in a rural community. *Ethiopian Medical Journal*, 13(1): 1–6.

Jermmott. J.B., Jermmot, L.S., Fong, G.T. and McCaffree, K. (1999). Reducing HIV risk-associated sexual behavior among African American Adolescents: Testing the generality of Intervention effects. *American Journal of Community Psychology*, 27(2): 161–187.

Kelly, J. et al. (1987). Stigmatization of AIDS patients by physicians. *American Journal of Public Health*, 77(7): 789–91.

Kelly, J.A., St. Lawrence, J.S., Smith, S. and Hood, H. (1987). Medical students attitudes towards AIDS and homosexual patients, *Journal of Medical Education*, 62(7): 549–556.

Kumar, A., Mehta, M., Badhan, S.K. and Gulati, N., (1997), Heterosexual Behavior and Condom Usage in an Urban Population of Delhi, India. *AIDS Care*, 9(3): 311–318.

Latting, J.K. (1990, Winter). Identifying the "isms": Enabling social work students to confront their biases, *Journal of Social Work Education*, 1: 36–44.

Lipson, J., and Brown, L. (1991). Do videotapes improve knowledge and attitudes about AIDS? *Journal of American College Health*, 39: 235–43.

Madden, T.J., Ellen, P.S. and Ajzen, I. (1992). A comparison of the theory of planned behavior and the theory of reasoned action. *Personality and Social Psychology Bulletin*, 18: 3–9.

Marcelo, R. (2003). *"AIDS could spin out of control in India,"* AIDS-INDIA Yahoogroups.com, 22 October, New Delhi.

Markova, I., McKee, K.J., Power, K. G. and Moodie E. (1995). The self and the other: Perception of the risk of HIV/AIDS in Scottish prisons, In Ivan Markova & Robert M. Farr (eds.) *Representation of Health, Illness and Handicap*, U.K. Harwood Academic Publishers: 111–29.

Mathai, R., Ross, M.W. and Hira, S. (1997). Concomitants of HIV/STD Risk Behaviors and Intention to Engage in Risk Behaviors in Adolescents in India. *AIDS Care*, 9(5): 563–575.

Melkote, S.R. and Goswami, D. (2000). Predictors of attitudes to persons with AIDS among young adults in India. *The Indian Journal of Social Work*, 61(1): 89–105.

Michael, R., Gagnon,J., Lanmann, E., and Kolata, G. (1994). *Sex in America*. New York: Little Brown & Company.

Moore, S.M., Rosenthal, D.A. (1991). Adolescent invulnerability and perception of AIDS risk. *Journal of Adolescent Research* 6: 164–

80. Nag, Moni. (1996). *Sexual Behavior and AIDS in India.* New Delhi: Vikas Publishing House.

Nath, M.B. (2000 March). Women's health and HIV: Experience from a sex workers' project in Calcutta. *Gender and Development,* 8(1):100–108.

National AIDS Control Organization (1997-98). *Country Scenario, New Delhi.*

National AIDS Control Organization (NACO) (2001). *National Baseline General Population Behavioral Surveillance Survey (BSS).* New Delhi: Ministry of Health and Family Welfare, Government of India.

National Intelligence Council (September 2002). *The Next Wave of HIV/AIDS: Nigeria, Ethiopia, Russia, India and China.* Washington D.C.

Neuman, L.W. (2000). *Social Research Methods, 4th ed.* Toronto, Ont.: Ally & Bacon.

Oakley, A., Fullerton, D. and Holland, J. (1995). Behavioral intervention for HIV/AIDS prevention. *AIDS,* 9(5): 479–86.

Owens, S. (1995). Attitudes toward and knowledge of AIDS among African American social work students, *Health and Social Work,* 20(2): 110–15.

Owens, S. (1992). Comfort and willingness of social work students to provide services to AIDS patients, *Journal of Teaching in Social Work,* 6(2): 99–113.

Panna L., Kumar, A., Ingle, G.K. and Gulati, N. (1998). Some AIDS-related issues and nursing students' willingness to provide aids care. *Journal of Communicable Diseases,* 30(1): 38–43.

Peterson, K. (1991). Social workers' knowledge about AIDS: A national survey, *Social Work,* 36(1): 31–7.

Potts, M. and Walsh, J. (2003). Tackling India's HIV Epidemic : Lessons from Africa. *British Medical Journal,* 326(21June): 1389–1392.

Reed, P., Wise, T. and Mann, L. (1984). Nurses' attitudes regarding Acquired Immunodeficiency Syndrome. *Nursing Forum,* 21(4) 153–56.

Richard, R., Van der and Pligt, J. (1991). Condom use among adolescents. *Journal of Community and Applied Social Psychology,* 1: 105–16.

Riley, J. and Greene, R. (1993). Influence of education on self perceived attitudes about HIV/AIDS among human services providers, *Social Work,* 38(4) 396–401.

Romer D., Black, M., Richardo, L., Feigelman, S., Kaljee, L., Galbraith, J., Nesbit, R., Hornik, R. and Stawton, B. (1994). Social influence on the sexual behavior of youth at risk for HIV exposure. *American Journal of Public Health,* 84: (6): 977–85.

Rotheram-Bonus, M., Reid, H., Rosario, M. and Kasen, S. (1995). Determinants of safer sex patterns among gay/bisexual male adolescents. *Journal of Adolescence,* 18: 3–15.

Slomin-Nevo, V., Ozawa, M. and Auslander, W. (1991). Knowledge, attitudes and behavior related to AIDS among youth in residential centers: Results from an exploratory study. *Journal of Adolescence,* 14: 17–33.

Rotherum-Bonus, M.J., Murphy, D.A., Fernandez, M.I. and Srinivasan, S. (1998). A brief HIV intervention for adolescent and young adults. *American Journal of Orthopsychiatry,* 68(4): 553–64.

Royse, D. and Birge, B. (1987). Homophobia and attitudes toward AIDS patients among medical, nursing and paramedical students, *psychological Report,* 61: 867–70.

Rubin, A. and Babbie, E. (2001). *Research Methods for Social Work,* 4th *ed.* Scarborough, Ont.: Thomas Learning.

Rubin, A., Johnson, P. and DeWeaver, K. (1996). Spring/Summer). Direct practice interests of MSW students: Changes from entry to graduation. *Journal of Social Work Education,* 2: 98–108.

Sachdev, P. (2002). *Sex, Lies and AIDS: Strategies for Preventions.* Seminar at India International Center, New Delhi, 6 April.

Sachdev, P. (1998). AIDS/HIV and university students in Delhi, India: Knowledge, beliefs, attitudes and behaviors, *Social Work in Health Care,* 26(4): 37–57.

Sachdev, P. (1997). Sex on campus: A preliminary study of knowledge, attitudes and behavior of university students in Delhi, India, *Journal of Biosocial Science,* 30: 95–105.

Sachdev, P. (1993). *Sex, Abortion and Unmarried Women.* Westport: CT: Greenwood Press.

Scalway, T. (2003). *Missing the Message? 20 Years of Learning From HIV/AIDS.* London, U.K: The Panos Institute.

Scollay, P., Doucett, M., Perry, M. and Winterbottom, B. (1992). AIDS education of college students: The effect of an HIV positive lecturer. *AIDS Education and Prevention,* 4: 16071.

Selvan, M.S., Ross, M.W., Kapadia, A.S., Mathai, R. and Hira, S. (2001). Study of Perceived Norms, beliefs and intended sexual behavior among higher secondary schools students in India. *AIDS Care,* 13(6): 779–788.

Sharma, V. and Sharma, A. (1997). Adolescent boys in Gujarat, India: their sexual behavior and their knowledge of acquired immunodeficiency syndrom and other sexually transmitted diseases. *Development and Behavioral Pediatrics*, 18: 399–404.

Shveller, J.A. and Pietersma, W.A. (2002). Preventing HIV/AIDS risk behavior among youth, *AIDS and Behavior*, 6(2): 123–29.

Silberman, J. (1991). The AIDS epidemic: Professional and personal concerns of graduate social work students in field placement, *Social Work in Health Care*, 15(3): 77–100.

Singh, Y. and Maliya, A. (1994). Long-distance truck drivers in India HIV-infection and their possible role in disseminating HIV in rural areas. *International Journal of STD and AIDS*, 5(2): 137–138.

Slonim-Nevo, V., Ozawa, M. and Auslander, W. (1991). Knowledge, attitudes and behavior related to AIDS among youth in residential centers: Results from an exploratory study. *Journal of Adolescence*, 14: 17–33.

Solomon, S., Kumaraswamy, N., Ganesh, A.K. and Amalraj, R. E. (1998). Prevalence and Risk Factors of HIV-1 and HIV-2 Infection in Urban and Rural Areas in Tamil Nadu, India, *International Journal of STD and AIDS*, 9(2): 98–103.

Stall, R. and McKusick, L. (1988). AIDS survey instrument. *Unpublished Instrument*, University of California, Center for AIDS Prevention Studies, San Francisco.

St. Lawrence, J.S., Jefferson, K.W., Alleyne, E. and Brasfield, T.L. (1995). Comparison of education vs. behavioral skills training interventions in lowering sexual HIV risk behavior of substance dependent adolescents. *Journal of Consulting Clinical Psychology*, 63: 154–57.

Temoshok, L., Sweet, D. and Zich, J. (1987). A three city comparison of the public's knowledge and attitudes about AIDS. *Psychological Health*, 1: 43–60.

UNAIDS, News. (2002). *Young People*, (January), p. 4.

UNAIDS. (2000). *Epidemiological fact sheet on HIV/AIDS and sexually transmitted infections by country*. Available www.unaids.org/hivaidsinfo/statistics/june00/fact.sheet/pdf/india/pdf

UNICEF cited in *Aiding Youth for Life*, 15 December, 2003: 1.

UNIFEM. (2003). *Gender and AIDS Web Portal*. 2 October.

United Nations Population Fund (UNFPA). (2002). *HIV Prevention Now*.Program Brief No. 4, February : 1–6.

United Nations Development Fund for Women (UNIFEM). (2003). *Gender and HIV/AIDS*, September 10: 1–2.

United Nations Population Fund (UNFPA). (2001). *HIV prevention now: An overview,* Program Brief No. 1, August: 1–6.

Van Servellen, G., Lewis, C. and Leke, B. (1988). Nurses' response to the AIDS crisis : Implications for continuing education program. *The Journal of Continuing Education in Nursing,* 19(1): 4–8.

VSO. (2003). *Gendering AIDS: Women, men, empowerment, mobilization. England, U.K.*

Walter H.L., Vaughan, R.D., Gladis, M.M., Regin, D.F., Kasen, S. and Cohall, A.T. (1992). Factors associated with AIDS risk behavior among high school students in an AIDS epicenter. *American Journal of Public Health,* 82(4): 528–32.

Watsa, M. (1994). *Youth: The sexual scenario in India.* Paper presented at the 3rd Asian Congress of Sexology. New Delhi, 27 November–2 December.

Waxler, S. (1989). Social welfare students and AIDS: A survey of knowledge, attitudes, and professional preparation. *Journal of Teaching in Social Work,* 3(1): 131–149.

Weiner, L. and Siegel, K. (1990). Social workers' comfort in providing services to AIDS patients, *Social Work* 35(January): 18–25.

Weisse, C., Turbiasz, A. and Whitney, D. (1995). Behavioral training and AIDS risk reduction: Overcoming barriers to condom use, In J. Edwards, R.S. Tindale, L. Heath, and E. J. Posavac (eds.) *Social Influence, Processes and Prevention,* 50–8. New York: Plenum Press.

Wisniewski, J.J. and Toomey, B.J. (1987). Are social workers homophobic? *Social Work,* 32: 454–55.

Yang, S. (2003). AIDS is India could become as dire as in Africa. *British Medical Journal,* 326: 1382–84.

Young, E. (1988). Nurses' attitude towards homosexuality: Analysis of change in Aids WORKSHOPS. *The Journal of Continuing Education in Nursing,* 19(1): 9-12.

Chapter 11

Women and Mental Health

Ashwani Kumar

Is there a gender difference? Is it just a myth that disproportionately more women suffer from mental health disorders because they are more frequently subject to social causes that lead to mental illness and psychosocial distress? NO. The Comparative analysis of empirical studies of mental disorders reveals a consistency across diverse societies and social contexts: symptoms of depression and anxiety as well as unspecified psychiatric disorder and psychological distress are more prevalent among women, whereas substance disorders are more prevalent among men. The disability-adjusted life years data recently tabulated by the World Bank reflect these differences. Depressive disorders account for close to 30 per cent of the disability from neuropsychiatric disorders among women, but only 12.6 per cent of that among men. Conversely, alcohol and drug dependence accounts for 31 per cent of neuro-psychiatric disability among men, but accounts for only 7 per cent of the disability among women. These patterns for depression and general psychological distress and substance disorders are consistently documented in many quantitative studies carried out in societies across the world (Desjarlais et al., 1995).

Epidemiologic and anthropological data point to different patterns and clusters of psychiatric disorders and psychological distress among women than among men. The origins of much of the pain and suffering particular to women can be traced to the social circumstances of many women's lives. Depression, hopelessness, exhaustion, anger and fear grow out of hunger, overwork, domestic and civil violence, entrapment and economic dependence. Understanding the sources of ill health for women means understanding how cultural and economic forces interact to undermine their social status.

Explanations proposed for gender differences in psychiatric morbidity in Asia, Africa, the Middle East and Latin America echo established associations among poverty, isolation and psychiatric morbidity for women in Western Europe and the United States (Dennerstein et al., 1993). In a now classic study by Brown and Harris (1978), depression was found to be more prevalent among working-class than middle-class women living in London. There is evidence that poor women experience more and more severe life events than the general population (Brown et al., 1975; Makosky, 1982); they are more likely to have to deal with chronic sources of social stress such as low quality housing and dangerous neighbourhoods (Makosky 1982; Pearlin and Johnson, 1977); they are at higher risk for becoming victims of violence (Belle, 1990; Merry 1981); and they are especially vulnerable to encountering problems in parenting and child care (Belle et al., 1990). Poverty also erodes intimate and other personal relationships (Cherlin, 1979; Wolf, 1987). In fact, social networks can represent additional stress for poor women as well as sources of support (Belle, 1990).) This gender difference has led some to contend that men tend to externalize their suffering through substance abuse and aggressive behaviour, resulting in an under-reporting of psychological distress. Women, in turn, more often suffer distress in the form of depression, anxiety, "nerves", and the like.

Ethnographic research and case descriptions enrich the quantitative findings of these prevalence studies of psychiatric morbidity, elaborating on the social context of depression, dependency and hopelessness and on the gendered dimension of these epidemiological clusters of social and psychological distress. Clusters appear as post-traumatic stress disorder and dissociative disorders, depression and sociopathy, and other mental illnesses which are highly correlated with societal breakdowns and social problems, such as civil strife, domestic violence, street violence, community disintegration, substance abuse, and family breakdown. Numerous case studies illustrate the configuration of such social psychological clusters. Das (1994), for example, recounts events in the life of an Indian woman following the loss of her husband and three sons in an ethnically charged riot, showing how her husband's family's subtle communication of the responsibility for the disaster converged with her own guilt to culminate in despair and eventual suicide. Links between economic hardship, child death, emotional deprivation, and psychological distress in women have also been documented in many anthropological studies, including recent work carried out in Brazil, Mexico and Pakistan.

Anthropology also offers an alternative approach to understanding the experience and expression of emotional distress. Complementing an epidemiological or clinical perspective with an ethnographic one, we find psychological pain realized not necessarily as "depression" or "anxiety" but in local idioms of distress—"nerves", "attacks", "heaviness of the heart" and intrusions by unwanted "spirits"—in studies carried out through South and North America, the Mediterranean region, Africa and Asia, and in Middle Eastern societies. Higher prevalence of such disorders is consistently found in females. Careful attention to social and cultural meanings associated with complaints of "nerves" often points to power conflicts, abuse and oppression in families and communities. Such findings appear in studies done in settings as diverse as Somalia, Iran, Malaysia, and among Central Americans who are refugees who fled civil strife and societal breakdown and currently live in the United States.

Poverty, domestic isolation, powerlessness (resulting, for example, from low levels of education and economic dependence), and patriarchal oppression are all associated with higher prevalence of psychiatric morbidity in women. In short, a considerable body of evidence points to the social origins of psychological distress for women. The effects of hunger, poverty and overwork, sexual and reproductive violence, domestic, civil and state violence, and the potential noxious effects of certain state economic policies, such as structural adjustment programmes and monetary crises have also been examined in the light of the mental health and general well-being of the majority of women. The conclusions from these reviews are indeed distressing. Malnutrition in many parts of the world is found more frequently among girls than boys. Manifesting sex bias is also found in traditional patterns of infanticide and newly practiced sex choices of foetuses, through selective abortion.

In the world of work, we find employment may bring self-esteem and independence; however, low paid or unpaid labour may contribute to oppression rather than independence. Many women work a "double day" maintaining households, raising children, carrying out economically productive activities in marketing and agriculture and in household-based industries. Numerous studies document that women "work" more hours than their husbands given their widely diverse economic and household responsibilities. Overwork may lead to exhaustion and stress. In addition, global and local traffic in women for commercial sex as well as household servitude entraps women, leading to high rates of mental illness. Sexual and reproductive violence, as well as rape during war, ethnic violence and civil strife, target women disproportionately. Severe and ongoing domestic violence has been documented in almost every country in the past decade; the World Bank (1993) estimates the consequences of familial and communal abuse account for approximately 5 per cent of the global burden of disease for women during the reproductive years. Such abuse is often associated with depression, dissociative disorders, and suicide.

It took the United Nation's "Decade for Women" to begin to make women's productive, as well as reproductive, roles visible to the world. Many development policies, and most recently in Asia, monetary policies to ease the debts of the rich and the consequent monetary crises, have hit women in traditional marketing, agricultural, and even in governmental and commercial sectors hard. Yet, the global consciousness-raising of the United Nations has spawned a number of programmes that enable women to be productive, to control their own labour, the means of production and their earnings. Programmes that are attuned to women's voices, needs, and hopes for the future for themselves and their families, and that contribute to women's control over economic and social/political resources have a direct and beneficial effect on women's mental health. They also have indirect effects, buffering women from oppressive conditions that place them at risk for mental illness and providing them the means to escape situations of violence, economic and sexual slavery and abuse.

Role of policies and programmes to address both the needs of the psychiatrically ill and the social origins of psychological and psychosocial distress

Such a description of the social origins underlying psychiatric disorders can be disheartening. However, the resilience of individuals and the ability of governments and community organizations to develop offer not only hope but examples as well.

Just as important is an understanding of the social origins of women's ill health is a recognition of what can be done and is being done to improve women's status and well-being. The development of policies and programmes consistent with broader definitions of health require listening to the women whom such programmes are designed to serve and giving voice to their concerns, at all stages of planning, implementation and management. Listening to women who will use and staff programmes maximizes the likelihood that services provided will fit well in local settings, and as a result be acceptable and used. The myth that poor women cannot or will not speak for themselves must be dispelled.

Much local listening work—that is, going into communities and talking with women about how they live and what their health and in particular mental health needs are—remains to be done. In the meantime, we may listen to the work of many

NGOs and women's groups that have mounted programmes to defend and promote the overall well-being of women, such as recent efforts being undertaken by Indonesian women's organizations to address the mental health consequences of the sexual violence perpetrated against Chinese Indonesian women during the May 1998 riots. NGOs and women's organizations are also seeking ways to give voice to ordinary women's concerns about feeding their families and caring for the sick in this stressful period created by the monetary crisis.

Building on local movements and enhancing grassroots strengths offer pathways through which the status of women and women's health may be improved. Numerous local initiatives abound, from adult literacy programmes in India to grassroots movements throughout the world's local communities of women, to resist oppression and to organize and reshape community health programmes.

The voices of the contributors to the 1991 National Council for International Health's Conference on Women's Health represent a broad perspective as well. Conference recommendations are directed toward women's overall empowerment; these include: *(i)* establishing baselines for women's health and well-being and measuring progress; *(ii)* developing ways of monitoring the impact of structural adjustment programmes on women's welfare, and establishing programmes to mitigate their adverse effects; *(iii)* enforcing or enacting legislation to improve women's status; *(iv)* addressing women's need for equitable employment and economic development; and (*v*) expanding education for women and girls.

Efforts at both the international and local levels are crucial, but to be maximally effective the two must connect. This may take several forms. One is the "listening" exercise mentioned above; exogenous donor agencies seeking to promote health and "development" should do so not only having listened but having given voice to the participants and intended beneficiaries of programmes. For women, this means being partners in the process of mainstreaming gender perspectives in health policy and development programmes. International support for local initiatives is another connecting mechanism. A third is learning from and using local programmes as models or creative inspiration for the designing of new initiatives.

Healthy Policies and Mental Health Policies

Health policies can be distinguished from "healthy" policies at the level of the state. Healthy policies are those government programmes which while not specifically aimed at fighting illness and disease, nonetheless have positive consequences for health. Healthy policies for women are supported by state gender ideologies that enhance the cultural, political and legal status of women by legitimizing equitable public investment and protection of females as well as males. Countries with equitable gender ideologies are far more likely to educate females at approximately the same rate as males and to provide women legal protection, political rights and economic opportunities, than countries that do not promote such equity. Although furthering gender equity in state ideologies requires the mobilization of political will and political action, as well as attention to women's voices and participation, the impact on women's well-being, and therefore the well-being of society, has been shown to be considerable.

Health policies that incorporate mental health into public health and address women's needs and concerns from childhood to old age can be developed in numerous ways to further mainstreaming of gender perspectives. Ethical considerations and competence of practitioners are central to the formulation of integrated health programs capable of redressing the trauma of rape, the stigma of sexual or domestic violence, the depression of isolation or gender oppression, and the anxiety of scarcity. One of the more troubling mental health consequences of general health status of communities is the effect on mothers of high infant and child mortality rates and high HIV infection rates affecting multiple family members across generations. Highly skilled clinicians as well as broader programmes are necessary to address the deeply troubling experiences women encounter when faced with decisions about how to make use of scarce family resources or how to plan for the care of children who may be orphaned because of familial HIV.

Although the social roots of many of these problems mean that they cannot simply be patched over with medical care, to ignore the potential role of the health care system to attend to needy women would imply that a society does not want to invest its resources in women's health. Institutions of health education, such as medical schools and training programmes for health workers, need to be evaluated and barriers to treating mental illness and the consequences of violence addressed. Communication among health workers, physicians, and women patients (and often men as well) is notoriously authoritarian in many places in the world, regardless of the sex of the physician or health worker, making a patient's disclosure of psychological distress or consequences of sexual violence difficult and at times stigmatized. Evaluation of training and enhancing the competence of primary care physicians and health workers to treat the consequences of domestic violence, sexual abuse and psychological distress and mental disorders may occur in tandem with a review of what women ideally want from health care givers.

International and state-sponsored health policies must also face the challenge of formulating moral but "culturally sensitive" responses to practices hazardous to the emotional and physical health of women and girls (such as female circumcision, female infanticide, gender-specific abortion, and feeding practices that discriminate against girl children). Such dilemmas can partially be resolved by offering support to local public health movements and grassroot efforts.

Health policies and accompanying programmes of health research may become leverage to mobilize political will and participation, and to promote change in policies controlled by other sectors of government. Continued documentation of the powerful relationship between the health of the whole society and female education is but one example. Evidence is overwhelming that the education of females is the single-most important factor in improving the health of infants and children, and of men. It is even a factor in reducing alcohol consumption by husbands (which, in turn, reduces male abusive behaviour). Similar analyses of links between legal inequities (such as gender discrimination in family and criminal law) and sexual and domestic violence and their health consequences for women and their families would provide one with another example. A third example is to emphasize the link between health and access to and control of economic resources and opportunities.

Health policies and "healthy" policies may both be fostered by and provide ways to encourage equitable state gender ideologies that bring about the mainstreaming of a gender perspective into the health sector. There are also several specific initiatives in the domain of mental health that call for concerted attention from the research community, international agencies, and local governments. The following recommendations do not propose formulas for the development of specific solutions, but suggest ways that recognize the complexities of creating mental health policies, and ultimately, mainstreaming a gender perspective in the health sector that recognizes the concerns of the very people most affected by the problems in question.

RECOMMENDATIONS FOR SPECIFIC INITIATIVES IN MENTAL HEALTH SERVICES AND TRAINING

• Upgrade the quality of mental health services

Mental health services have a crucial role to play in alleviating suffering associated with psychiatric illnesses, emotional distress, psychological disorders, and behavioural pathology. Abused women, troubled children, those traumatized by political violence, those who have attempted suicide or are addicted to alcohol or narcotics, and especially those who suffer acute or chronic mental illnesses can be helped substantially by competent mental health care. We have seen how women suffer disproportionately from mental illnesses such as depression and anxiety, and dissociative disorders associated with sexual abuse, and yet these are the illnesses that competent clinicians may best help. With recent advances in psychiatric medications and specialized forms of psycho-social interventions, the potential for benefit is greater than at any time in history.

Yet mental health services in most societies are inadequate. Well-trained practitioners are scarce, drugs and psycho-social interventions are unavailable or of poor quality, and even where expertise and resources exist, they seldom reach into the communities where the needs are greatest. The human rights of the mentally ill are often severely compromised, and mental health care is too often associated with abusive social control. Financial investment is required for sustainable programmes, and creativity is needed to build programmes that join local resources with professional knowledge.

Mainstreaming a gender perspective in the mental health sector—through educating women at all levels of society about the possibilities of mental health interventions and the potential for services and programmes—is central to the success of mental health programme development. The development of community-based programmes may build upon the engagement of many women to their local communities and their commitment to community and family health. Formal mental health services, including rational drug policies for psychotropic medications and the reliable provision of adequate supplies at reasonable costs (selected generic anti-depressants, anti-psychotic and anti-convulsant drugs), must be complemented by non-medical support groups, consumer groups and healing institutions that provide crucial care in many communities.

- **Encourage systematic efforts to upgrade the amount and quality of mental health training for workers at all levels, from medical students to graduate physicians, from nurses to community health workers**

Essential to mental health programmes is a small cadre of well-trained mental health professionals: psychiatrists, psychologists, social workers and psychiatric nurses. They are the ones who must lead efforts to establish priorities of mental health in medical education and health policy. Training primary care physicians, nurses and health workers in the recognition and appropriate referral and/or treatment of mental illness is central to expanding community services to meet needs. Specific training in diagnosis and management of psychiatric conditions is required to improve the quality of mental health services offered in primary care. And since community practitioners often depend almost exclusively on agents of pharmaceutical companies for new information on medications, initiatives in continuing education are needed to provide more basic training in the safe and effective use of psychotropic medications.

With appropriate training and supervision, non-physician primary health workers can learn to diagnose, treat, and organize follow-up programmes for a substantial fraction of cases of depression, anxiety and epilepsy, and can, with appropriate supervision, manage patients with chronic schizophrenia in the community if their social welfare is provided. WHO has developed training programmes and shown they can be effectively employed in societies as diverse as India, the Philippines, and Tanzania. In societies in which non-physicians provide a substantial portion of primary care, specialized training activities are a cost-effective means of improving and extending mental health services.

Mainstreaming a gender perspective may build on the interests of many women professionals who have entered the field of mental health care as psychiatrists, psychiatric nurses, counselors and social workers.

• Promote efforts to improve state gender policies, toward interdicting violence against women, and toward empowering women economically, and to make women central in policy planning and implementation of mental health services. Research should evaluate the mental health consequences of these programmes for women, for children, and for men

As we have noted above, investing in the health, education, and well-being of women is of high priority for improving the mental health of populations in low and middle-income countries. The World Bank's 1993 World Development Report clearly demonstrates that educating women to primary school level is the single most important determinant of both their own and their children's health. Women's education is an equally valuable investment for the mental health of women, men and children. Such education also renders women less likely to tolerate domestic violence and abuse, or the spending of substantial portions of the family income on drinking or gambling by their spouses. Educated women are also more likely to be receptive to and engaged, as equal partners, in public health programmes.

Women throughout the world constitute the vast majority of caretakers of first and last resort for chronically disabled family members, including mentally retarded children, demented elderly, and adults suffering a major mental illness. Minimally, it is in a community's long-term social interest to assist with this burden through formal health services. In addition, because women are critical to the success of health policies, their participation in formulating mental health policies should be encouraged, with governments, international organizations and NGOs defining avenues for women to exercise leadership roles. Policies may be evaluated by women's groups not only in terms of how they support women's mental health but also in terms of the quality of services offered to women, children and men.

- **Encourage initiatives to attend to the causes and consequences of collective and interpersonal violence**

Collective and interpersonal violence is one of the most pressing problems in the world today. Wars, prolonged conflicts, ethnic strife, and political repression lead to deep trauma and psychological problems that persist beyond the period of conflict and violence. While only profound changes in international and national politics will reduce armed conflicts, peace and security initiatives should be strongly encouraged. In addition, mental health concerns should be more widely understood in peace and security programmes. For ethnic conflict, for instance, mental health issues—from the effect of racism on ethnic identity to the vicious cycles of revenge—should become the target of new policies, such as education in schools. Transnational initiatives to treat trauma may assist in modest but effective ways as well as to quickly respond to and aid victims of collective violence. Intervention programmes of therapy and triage, which have been shown to have beneficial effects, need to be supported internationally as well as locally given costs and limited services in many parts of the world. Women's organizations have taken major roles in leading such efforts in the past and can be models for future efforts as well.

Curtailing and preventing interpersonal and domestic violence (often generated by community violence and breakdown) requires the mainstreaming of a gender perspective to formulate policies both in health care services and in the legal system. Although medical care for physical wounds and mental health care for psychological wounds may mitigate long-term suffering, deterrence and ultimately prevention require laws that make domestic violence against women (and children) a crime.

- **Direct efforts specific to primary prevention of mental disorders, and behavioural, psychosocial and neurological disorders**

Such efforts would survey the scientific knowledge base, examine primary prevention activities around the world, address the cross-cultural relevance of prevention programmes, and define training needs and related activities. Successful prevention programmes call for the integration of biological and psychosocial factors, and the active promotion of proven preventive programmes. Models taking account of the co-morbidity of many disorders, the clusters of psychiatric disorders and psychosocial distress, must be developed in order to encourage interventions to support individuals who are afflicted with mental illness. In addition, prevention programmes require an understanding of indigenous protective factors, such as the activities of caretakers of those who are ill and those local practices that enhance the mental and physical health and well-being of individuals and of communities. Listening to women professionals and laymen should help in identifying these factors.

CONCLUSION

If the goal of improving women's well-being from childhood through old age is to be achieved, "healthy" policies aimed at improving the social status of women are needed along with the "health policies" targeting the entire spectrum of women's health needs. Such an emphasis calls for state gender ideologies that encourage investment in women's health in broad ways, from education to economic empowerment and through legal and political mechanisms that enhance the status of women. It also calls for a concerted effort to improve and enhance social and mental health services and the competence of professionals and programmes in concert with the improvement of health services overall.

REFERENCES

Angell, M. (1997). The Ethics of Clinical Research in the Third World. [Editorial] *New England Journal of Medicine,* 337(12): 847–849.

Belle, D. (1990). Poverty and Women's Mental Health. *American Psychologist,* 45: 385–389.

Belle, D., Dill, D., Longfellow, C. and Makosky, V. (1990). Stressful Life Conditions and Mental Health of Mothers. In *Women and Depression: Research Gaps and Priorities.* Symposium presented at the Annual Meeting of the American Psychological Association, Atlanta, Georgia (August).

Boddy, J. (1989). Wombs and Alien Spirits: Women, Men, and the Zar Cult in Northern Sudan. Madison, WI: University of Wisconsin Press.

Brown, G.W., Bhrolchain, M. and Harris, T. (1975). Social Class and Psychiatric Disturbance among Women in an Urban Population. *Sociology,* 9: 225–257.

Brown, G. W. and Harris, T. O. (1978). Social Origins of Depression: A Study of Psychiatric Disorder in Women. New York: The Free Press.

Cherlin, A. (1979). Work Life and Marital Dissolution. In *Divorce and Separation: Context, Causes and Consequences,* edited by G. Levenger and O. Moles, 156–166. New York: Basic Books.

Cohen, A. (1997). Site Visits. Updates on Global Mental and Social Health 2:1.

Das, V. (1994). Moral Orientations to Suffering: Legitimation, Power and Healing. In *Health and Social Change in International Perspective*, edited by L. Chen, A. Kleinman and N. Ware, pp 139–170. Boston: Harvard Series on Population and International Health.

Davis, D.L. and Low, S.M., (Ed.) (1989). *Gender, Health and Illness: The Case of Nerves.* New York: Hemisphere Publishing.

Dennerstein, L., Asbury, J. and Morse, C. (1993). *Psychosocial and Mental Health Aspects of Women's Health.* Geneva: World Health Organization.

Desjarlais, R., Kleinman, A., Eisenberg, L. and Good, B. (1995). *World Mental Health: Problems, Priorities, and Responses in Low-Income Countries:* Oxford University Press.

Farias, P. (1991). Emotional Distress and its Socio-Political Correlates in Salvadoran Refugees: Analysis of a Clinical Sample. *Culture, Medicine and Society*, 15: 167–192.

Finkler, K. (1985). Symptomatic Differences between the Sexes in Rural Mexico. *Culture, Medicine and Psychiatry*, 9: 27–57.

Good, B. and Good, M-J. D. (1982). Toward a Meaning Centered Analysis of Popular Illness Categories: "Fright Illness" and "Heart Distress" in Iran. In *Cultural Conceptions of Mental Health and Therapy*, edited by A. Marsella and G. White, 141-166. Dordrecht: Reidel.

Jacobson, J. (1993). Women's Health: The Price of Poverty. In *The Health of Women: A Global Perspective*, edited by M. Koblinsky, J. Timyan, and J. Gay, 3–32. Boulder, CO: Westview Press.

Koblinsky, M, Timyan, J. and Gay, J. (Ed.) (1993). *The Health of Women: A Global Perspective.* Boulder, CO: Westview Press.

Lewis, I.M. (1986). *Religion in Context: Cults and Charismas.* Cambridge: Cambridge University Press.

Lurie, P. and Wolfe, S.M. (1997). Unethical Trials of Interventions to Reduce Prenatal Transmission of the Human Immunodeficiency Virus in Developing Countries. [Editorial] *New England Journal of Medicine*, 337(12): 853–856.

Makosky, V. (1982). Sources of Stress: Events or Conditions? In *Lives in Stress: Women and Depression*, edited by D. Belle, 35–53. Beverly Hills, CA: Sage Publications.

Malik, I.A., Bukhtiari, N., Good, M.J.D. (1992). Mothers' Fear of Child Death: A Study in Urban and Rural Communities in Northern Punjab, Pakistan. *Social Science and Medicine*, 35: 1043–1053.

Merry, S. (1981). *Urban Danger*. Philadelphia: Temple University Press.

Msamanga, G.I. and Fawzi, W.W. (1997). The Double Burden of HIV Infection and Tuberculosis in Sub-Saharan Africa. [Editorial; Comment] *New England Journal of Medicine* 337(12): 849–851.

Naeem, S. (1992). Vulnerability Factors for Depression in Pakistani Women. *Journal of the Pakistan Medical Association,* June:137–138.

Nations, M.K. and Rebhun, L. (1988). Angels with Wet Wings Won't Fly: Maternal Sentiment in Brazil and the Image of Neglect. Culture, *Medicine and Psychiatry,* 12:171–200.

Ong, A. (1987). *Spirits of Resistance and Capitalist Discipline: Factory Women in Malaysia.* Albany: State University of New York Press.

Pearlin, L.I. and Johnson, J.S. (1977). Marital Status, Life-Strains and Depression. *American Sociological Review,* 82: 652–663.

Rosenfield, A. and Maine, D. (1985). Maternal Mortality—A Neglected Tragedy. Where Is the "M" in MCH? *The Lancet,* 2(8446): 83–85.

Scheper-Hughes, N. (1987). Culture, Scarcity and maternal Thinking: Mother Love and Child Death in Northeast Brazil. In *Child Survival,* edited by N. Scheper-Hughes, pp. 187–208. Dordrecht: Reidel.

Scheper-Hughes, N. (1992). *Death without Weeping: The Violence of Everyday Life in Brazil.* Berkeley: University of California Press.

Scheper-Hughes, N. (1995). The Primacy of the Ethical: Propositions for a Militant Anthropology.(Objectivity and Militancy: A Debate) *Current Anthropology,* 36(3): 409–421.

Whalen, C.C. et al. (1997). A Trial of Three Regimens to Prevent Tuberculosis in Ugandan Adults Infected with the Human Immuno-deficiency Virus. *New England Journal of Medicine* 337(12): 801–808.

Ware, N. and Good, M-J.D. (1995). Women. In *World Mental Health: Problems, Priorities, and Responses in Low-Income Countries.* Edited by Robert Desjarlais, Arthur Kleinman, Leon Eisenberg, and Byron Good. Oxford University Press. 179–206.

Wolf, B. (1987). Low-Income Mothers at Risk: The Psychological Effects of Poverty-Related Stress. Unpublished dissertation, Harvard Graduate School of Education, Cambridge, MA.

World Bank. (1993). *World Development Report : Investing in Health.* New York: Oxford University Press.

Chapter 12

Women and Leprosy

Harvinder Kaur

Until recently, the inter-relationships among gender, health and disease have received little attention. With the exception of pregnancy and the reproductive period, it is assumed that the sequel of infection and disease are similar for men and women. So, uniform approaches to treatment and disease control are adopted. However, in the last few years, important gender differences in the impact of diseases such as cardiac disease, cancer and mental illness have emerged (Stacey and Olesen, 1993. Herman, 1992; Verbrugge, 1985). Women have higher rates for most non-fatal chronic conditions. Non-fatal conditions accumulate over time and women end up with more chronic conditions on the average than same aged men. In developing countries, communicable diseases, together with illnesses relating to childbirth, account for most morbidity in women (World Bank, 1993). In the developed world too, women are sicker than men. Doyal (1995) explains that while women risk contracting the same endemic disease as men, both biological and social factors may increase exposure or worsen the effects. In India, females below the age of 30 have higher death rates from illness than men in the same age group (BMJ, 1996). The poor health status is a major cause of India's female deficient sex ratio. Cultural factors, gender bias and inadequate health care and the contributing factors to women's poor health. Women in India experience more episodes of illness than men and are less likely to receive medical treatment before the illness is well advanced. Differences in the utilization of healthcare facilities and other aspects of treatment seeking behaviour between men and women have become evident. It is reported that men avail of the opportunity to report their ill-health (Leslie and Rao Gupta, 1989; Ettling, 1989, Finerman, 1989, Cosminsky, 1987; Balijaev, 1986). WHO (1995) note that in the developing world, women use health services less than men. High proportions of women receive no treatment for their illness; for those who do, the most common treatment methods entail self care, home remedies, or traditional medicine (BMJ, 1996).

Research on gender differences in tropical diseases like leprosy is limited. Studies done so far reflect that leprosy affects women less commonly than men at majority of places (Ulrich, 1993; Misra and Ramesh, 1987; Noordeen, 1985, Mahapatro, 1984, Pearson, 1982, Job and Selvapandian, (1978). This could be due to under reporting in females because they are less mobile in the community (Pearson, 1982). Sometimes, traditions prevent their coming forward for clinical examination and diagnosis. This is exemplified by the practice of 'purdah' among the women in Pakistan (Mull, 1989). They are found to come when the disease is advanced (Nakai, 1980).

Some beliefs regarding the cause of the disease are linked to gender-related stereotypes. It has been noted that women are less likely to undergo complete physical examinations by male personnel (Pearson, 1982; Mull, 1989). Even after identifying the symptoms, women have been observed to depend exclusively on non-medical treatment for longer period in comparison to men (Rao, 1996).

The present study is an attempt to look into the nature of problems faced by women leprosy patients in terms of social, cultural, psychological and economic onslaughts which hamper them in utilizing health care facilities.

METHODOLOGY

The present study is based in Delhi, the National Capital, which is considered to be a low endemic area for leprosy. It is estimated that the city has 8,690 leprosy cases, with the prevalence rate of 5 per 10,000 population (NLEP 1994). Under the National Leprosy Eradication Programme (NLEP), treatment and other modes of patient care are provided through 12 hospitals, including 9 government and 3 non-government treatment centres.

In order to get the representative sample from Delhi, 2 government and 2 private/non-governmental hospitals were selected amongst 12 hospitals for study. The selection was based on their annual case load and geographical location in the city. The study is related to women leprosy patients (above 15 years of age) seeking treatment from Safdarjung Hospital, Dr. Ram Manohar Lohia Hospital, The Leprosy Mission Hospital and Skin Institute. The government-run Safdarjung Hospital and Dr. Ram Monohar Lohia Hospital receive maximum number of leprosy patients from all parts of Delhi. The Leprosy Mission Hospital and Skin Institute are amongst the three non-governmental hospitals associated with leprosy control in Delhi. The hospital records between the year 1991 to 1994 suggest that on an average, 383 new leprosy patients reported for treatment in hospital out of which 53 were women from Delhi. This ratio is too low to that reported in different studies (Ulrich, 1993; Misra and Ramesh, 1987; Noordeen 1985, Mahapatro, 1984; Pearson, 1982; Job and Selvapandian, 1987). Hence, this study represents the findings of those motivated treatment seekers who could reach the hospital.

The data were collected using interview schedules which had both structured questions to collect quantitative data and open-ended unstructured questions to collect qualitative information. The interview schedule was pretested on ten patients and the required modifications were made. In one year time (from 14 March 1995 to 24 February 1996), all the women leprosy patients, irrespective of the type of leprosy, paucibacillary (PB) or multibacillary (MB), above 15 years of age, living in Delhi and have undergone minimum three months of treatment from the concerned hospital, were taken. It has been assumed that in three months of treatment, patients would know about their disease and would be able to communicate their experiences. After taking patient's consent, home visits were made and patients were interviewed at their residence. In all, 160 patients could be interviewed.

All the women leprosy patients approached, agreed to a participate in the study and welcomed the researcher during home visits, except for one, who hesitated as she had kept her disease secret from others. The present paper is a qualitative presentation of issues using case illustrations. Patients' names have been changed to conceal their identity.

RESULTS

Utilisation of Health Care Facilities

The utilization pattern of health care facilities, in the present case, leprosy treatment by female patients, has been studied. In order to understand the complexities faced by the women patients, each aspect is explained by the case illustration.

Treatment compliance

Being a chronic disease with long treatment schedules, it becomes difficult to maintain the desired compliance of patients. The major hurdles reported by them are economic constraints, long distance to the hospital, dependency on others to be escorted and household work responsibilities. Fifty-one women in the present study were accompanied by their husbands to the hospital and thirty eight by other family members. These treatment hurdles hampered patients like Shahnaz Begum (Illustration I) to continue her treatment regularly:

Illustration I : Shahnaz, 30, belonged to a low socio-economic, uneducated, joint family. About a year back, when she developed pain in her limbs, her husband brought her to the hospital where she was put on anti-leprosy treatment. She had anaesthetic hands and feet (GSA), which made her prone to injuries and burns. She often used to get fever and joint pain due to Type II reaction (one of the complexities of leprosy).

Being in a joint family, she had a heavy domestic responsibilities. More than this, the ignorant and demanding attitude of her in-laws caused difficulties for her to carry on her life with leprosy. She could hardly take rest, even during fever or severe joint pain.

They were living almost 30 kilometres away from the hospital and she was dependent on her husband in order to visit the hospital. Her husband was an unskilled labourer on daily wages. So in order to save wage loss, he could not take her to the hospital regularly. Moreover, they found travelling to be expensive, every trip cost them about Rs. 50. As a result, she was unable to continue her treatment on a regular basis.

But there are other real hurdles too that are not felt by the affected. These include the social stigma attached to the disease, ignorance towards the importance of its treatment and the status of women. It can be understood by the following case illustration of Enami Devi.

Illustration II : Enami Devi, 20 belonged to a lower socio-economic status family. Because of her disease and the related reactions, she was not able to carry out household chores. As a result, her mother-in-law used to abuse her. Due to lack of education, the family failed to realise the importance of treatment, although they were well aware of her disease.

Enami was married for a year. Her parents-in-law expected her to bear a child but she had a spontaneous abortion. Due to weakness and the disease, she was advised to postpone pregnancy till she was fully cured. But her in-laws, including her husband, did not understand this and continued to pressurize her to bear a child. Since there were no leprosy-related deformities, she did not face any stigma. Due to lack of motivation to get her treated, nobody accompanied her to the hospital. As a result, she was taking her treatment irregularly. Her condition deteriorated due to irregularity in treatment. But sometimes the ignorance and prevalent beliefs can be hazardous. Poonam's case (Illustration III) demonstrates this.

Illustration III : Poonam, 20, got married in a joint family. Most of the family members, including herself, were illiterate. She was having hypo pigmented patches and anaesthesia over her right arm since the last 9 years. But it was not diagnosed till she came to the hospital some 4 months' back.

During the period without treatment, she followed

suggestions that were given to her by others. She had consulted a private practitioner who diagnosed it to be some sort of skin rash. The treatment was not effective. After marriage, at her in-law's place, she was advised to burn the patch with acid. Poonam followed the advice. Her skin got severely burned and infected, although, because of anaesthesia, she could not feel the pain. The wound healed, leaving behind a big scar over her forearm.

Surgical correction of deformities

Facilities for reconstructive surgery are most accessible in Leprosy Mission Hospital which is also a referral centre for the same. The surgery for leprosy patients in performed free of cost. Patient's motivation to undergo reconstructive surgery has been studied among the patients with flexible deformity. It was found that 16 of the 25 (64%) patients with flexible deformity have enquired about the possibility of correcting deformities. After counselling, 19 (76%) of then agreed to undergo surgery. Five of them actually got operated. Three (12%) refused and another three (12%) desired to take prior permission of their husband. The main reason for hesitation was the need of hospitalisation that might reveal their disease that could otherwise be concealed. Another reason cited was their inability to escape from domestic chores. Renu's experience is illustrative (Illustation IV).

Illustration IV: Renu, 25, noticed her hands getting anaesthetic and started her treatment in the hospital. Knowing that she had leprosy, out of the fear of social rejection, she kept the diagnosis to herself. While cooking, she often got burnt in her anaesthetic hand. Gradually she also developed claw hand deformity. All through her treatment, she was encouraged to perform physiotherapy exercises to keep her claw hand flexible and joints supple. Although she completed her therapy, the deformity remained. She was advised reconstructive surgery that needed admission to hospital. It was not easy for her without her husband's permission. She was afraid that it would bring her disease to her husband's knowledge.

Her apprehension was justified because when he came to

know that she had leprosy, he segregated her from the children and also decided to send her to her parents. He believed that leprosy can never be cured and that it is a hereditary disease.

In this case, the social worker intervened to solve the matter and helped the husband to understand the disease and also convinced him that Renu was completely cured of the disease. However, there may be many such cases who suffer in silence because of the prevalent beliefs in the society

Treatment pathways followed by patients

In order to understand the treatment-seeking problems, the treatment pathways followed by the patients before they reach the sampled hospitals for anti-leprosy treatment, has been studied. A flow chart of each patient's treatment pathway was prepared. It has been found that the patients have gone through a long route to the hospital. The general trend followed by them shows that once aware of the symptoms, they consult the local private practitioners (qualified allopathic practitioners), alternate medicine practitioners (homeopathic, ayurvedic and unani practitioners), quacks (unqualified doctors) or traditional healers (*vaid, hakeem*), whom they were more familiar with. If they were not satisfied with the treatment received, they would come to Delhi to seek treatment. Delhi is preferred mainly by those who had somebody known in the city.

In the present study, 54 (33.75%) patients approached hospitals when the symptom emerged. Thirty-one (19.37%) of them approached the sampled hospitals directly, at different intervals of time. Among the rest, 90 (56.25%) patients had paid a visit to the private practitioners. Seventeen (10.62%) patients who had either been to traditional healers, local quacks or preferred self treatment. But five (3.12%) patients believing that leprosy is God's curse, opted for 'religious' or 'ritual' treatment ('puja' or *jhadhphoonk*). Since 106 (66.25%) patients had consulted more than one treatment practitioner, there is overlapping of data. On an average each patient had visited more than two treatment centres before they reached the hospital. The maximum number of institutions visited by certain patients were 11. The importance of creating awareness of the disease and its treatment facilities can be understood from the case illustration of Nazma (Illustration V). She not only had spent ten precious years of her life hunting for leprosy treatment, but also lost her fingers and toes in the process, because of lack of proper treatment.

Illustration V: Nazma, 34, had spent half of her life with leprosy and its deformities. It took her almost a decade to reach the hospital. It all started after two years of her marriage during their stay in the village, when hypo pigmented patches appeared over her legs. Her family mistook them for some skin changes and ignored the problem for 3–4 years. Then she started getting blisters/boils over her hands and feet. Her family took them for burns initially, but she continued getting them repeatedly. Then they opted for *'jhadh-phoonk'* in the village temple. In the temple, she was provided with *'dhoop-raakh'* (incense ash collected from the temple) to be applied on boils. This weekly practice was followed for almost one year. This was because the boils used to get healed.

Then the couple moved to Delhi where they consulted a private practitioner. She was repeatedly getting ulcers. During one of her visits to their local dispensary for ulcer management, she was advised about leprosy treatment in the hospital. As she was suffering too much, she immediately went to the hospital where anti-leprosy treatment was finally started. In the absence of timely treatment and care, the patient had developed multiple grade III irreversible deformities. Her fingers and toes got defused.

Treatment gap and its reasons

Since the symptoms of leprosy are vague and awareness in the general public is low, many people do not come for appropriate treatment at an early stage. Treatment gap is also caused due to ignorance and long treatment pathways followed. In the present study, anti-leprosy treatment for more than 24 per cent patients was started within six months of developing symptoms, for more than 9 per cent within one year, while in more than 37 per cent, treatment gap, i.e., gap between their first symptoms noticed and the start of treatment, is more than three years. Nazma (Illustration V) is one of such cases.

The reasons for this treatment gap were explored. Among the most commonly reported reasons stated by 48 patients, was that they were taking treatment elsewhere before coming to the proper centre. The earlier consultants included various private practitioners, alternative medicine practitioners and local quacks who could not diagnose their disease and guide patients to get appropriate treatment. Thirty-four patients did not find their symptoms harmful enough to warrant any treatment. In patients, symptoms were not obvious enough to motivate them to go for treatment, as has been observed in case of Nazma (Illustration V). Four patients could not take treatment due to non-availability of treatment facilities in their locality. Three women remained untreated in the absence of an escort to take them to the hospital. Due to economic constraints, one patient postponed her treatment. Personal reasons and problems too hindered treatment seeking.

Among the first symptoms noticed by the patients, hypo pigmented patches motivated 25 (27.7%) of the 90 patients to come for early treatment within one year of noticing the symptoms. Anaesthesia made 17(36.95%) of the 46 women to come for early treatment. Pain in the joints motivated six (60%) of the 10 patients to report for treatment within one year. Four of the six patients (66.66%) who had swelling in the limbs reported for treatment within six months.

DISCUSSION

Recently, gender-related studies have come to the forefront. Gender-specific data are essential, not only to assure that women are being reached, but to assure that resources are equitably and effectively shared. Women do not deserve less, but society, culture and tradition often block their access to what is rightfully theirs. Although female mortality and morbidity are the gross indicators of women's health, the quality of their lives is an indicator of their ability to develop and maximize their potential. Women must be empowered by training, education and participation to seek prevention and treatment of diseases which may kill them. The elements required for women to have effective access to care are myriad and complex. While ensuring the availability of facilities and personnel within reasonable distance is indeed a primary requirement. Effective access to care can only be ensured if that care is considered affordable, appropriate and acceptable by the women it aims to serve. The 19th International Health Conference of the National Council of International Health, held in Arlington, Virginia in June 1991 on the theme "Women's Health: The Action Agenda for the 1990s" was notable for highlighting the complexity of issues that restrict women's access to care, many of which relate to demand rather than supply. To be sure, factors such as distance from the site of care, lack of availability of equipment and supplies at the site, and lack of money to cover the costs of transportation and treatment were mentioned. The key constraints to access were identified as being of a socio cultural or informational nature, including lack of awareness of health issues, the low social and legal status assigned to women in most cultures, lack of self-esteem and sense of control, religious restriction, and perceived inappropriateness of care.

Women's lack of knowledge and awareness, which can range from not knowing the location of a health care delivery side to a lack of understanding of the danger signs or gravity of a condition, have a profound impact on health care utilization. Often women do not perceive themselves as having a problem or of being at risk. In addition, particular conditions may not be associated with a need for care, particularly care from the formal system. A condition may be so prominent in the community, or the woman may have suffered its symptoms for so long, that it is not recognised as problematic. Moreover, the cultural barriers and the limitations of taking decisions to seek treatment/health care by the women further hamper the utilization of health care facilities.

Recognition of the fact that they (women) need treatment intervention is as important as continuing the treatment. It becomes more important in the case of leprosy where the treatment is long and there are various aspects of self care to prevent deformities and disabilities. Although efforts are being made to reduce the treatment duration and simplifying the treatment process to make it more and more accessible and acceptable. It is not a question of the health system's supply of services, rather, how well women are able to utilise these services.

Recommendations

- Recognising the effects of cultural and familial restrictions on women's mobility, as well as lack of awareness of the need for care and signs of danger or potential problems.
- Exploring and evaluating creative ways to bring services closer to women.
- Overcoming informational barriers by increasing women's knowledge and understanding of the need for and availability of care, the risks they face, symptoms of illness and signs of danger. Also making them aware of their right to be healthy and not in pain or exhausted.
- Providing women with education and leadership training to enhance their sense of self-worth, improving their self-esteem and their right to good health.
- Reaching the decision makers, like the husband, father and or mother-in-law, to enhance women in seeking health care.
- Overcoming the cultural barriers through health education by recognizing the conflict between modern medicine and traditional explanations for health phenomenon.

REFERENCES

Baljaev, A.E., Sharma, G.K., Brohult, J.A. and Haque, M.A. (1986). Studies on the detection of malaria at Primary Health Centers. Part II. Age and sex composition of patients subjected to blood examination in passive case detection. *Indian Journal Malaria* 23 (19).

British Medical Journal. (1996). News: India's women get poor deal on health care, says World Bank, 312, 1627–1628.

Cosminsky, S. (1987). "Women and health care on a Guatemalan plantation." *Social Science Medicines*, 25: 1163.

Doyal, L. (1995). *What makes women sick: gender and the political economy of health*. London: Macmillan.

Ettling, M.B., T. Krongthong S., Krachaklin and Bualombai, P. (1989). "Evaluation of malaria clinics in Maesot, Thailand: use of serology to assess coverage." Transactions of the Royal Society of Tropical Medicine and Hygiene, 83, 325.

Finerman, R. (1989). Who benefits from health-care decisions? Family medicine in an Andean Indian community" in: *What we know about health transition:* The cultural, social and behavioural determinants of health. Health Transition Series, 2 (II), 657, Canberra.

Herman R. (1992). "What doctors don't know about women: a special report." *Washington Post* (Health) December.

Job C.K. and Selvapandian A.J. (1978). Leprosy: Diagnosis and Management. Hind Kusht Nivaran Sangh, p. 7.

Leslie, J. and Gupta, G.R. (1989). "Utilization of formal services for maternal nutrition and health care in the third world." Washington, DC : International Center for Research on Women.

Mahapatro, B. (1984). Epidemiology: endemicity of leprosy in rural health center. The XII Internal Leprosy Congress, New Delhi.

Misra, R. S. and Ramesh V. (1987). Leprosy in the Union Territory of Delhi. *Indian Journal Leprosy*, 59, 293–299.

Mull, J.D., Shear, W. C, Gans, L. P. and Mull, D. S. (1989). Culture and 'compliance' among leprosy patients in Pakistan. *Social Science Medicines*, 29(7), 199–811.

Nakai E. (1980). Leprosy in Northen India—an epidemiological study in Ghatempur Block. Japanese *Journal of Leprosy*, 49, 77–86.

NLEP. (1994). National Leprosy Eradication Programme in India. Guidelines for multidrug treatment in non-endemic districts. Leprosy Division, Directorate General of Health Services (DGHS), Ministry of Health and Family Welfare, New Delhi.

Noordeen, S.K. (1985). The epidemiology of leprosy. In: Leprosy (Hasting RC Ed.) Churchil Livingstone Publishers, Edinburg, 15–30.

Pearson, M. (1982). Social factors and leprosy in Lamjung, West Central Nepal: implication for disease control. *Ecology of Disease*, 1(4), 229–236.

Roa, S., Garole, V., Walawalkar, S., Khot, S. and Karandikar N. (1996).

Gender differentials in the social impact of leprosy. *Leprosy Review*, 67, 190–199.

Stacey, M. and Olesen, V. (1993). "Women, Men and Health." (special issue), *Social Science Medical*, 36 (1).

Ulrich, M., Zulueta, A.M., Dittmar, G.C., Sampson, C., Pinardi, A.M., Rada, E.M. and Aranzazu N. (1993). Leprosy in women: Characteristics and Repercussions. *Social Science Medicines*, 37 (4), 445–456.

Verbrugge, L.M. (1985). "Gender and health: an update on hypotheses and evidence." *Journal Health and Social Behaviour* 26; 156–182.

World Bank. (1993). World Development Report—investing in health. New York: Oxford University Press.

WHO. (1995). "Women's health: improve our health, improve the world." Geneva: WHO.

Seminar Report

The Constitution of India is one of the most comprehensive documents written by any country. It ensures to govern its people with justice and equality. One major beneficiary group of the Constitution is women, who legally have equal rights to participate in the political and social processes of the country. However, the Constitutional provision in itself cannot empower women. The status of around 500 million women and girls who compose slightly less than half of India's population and around one-sixth of all the world's female people has remained low and depressed.

One of the commitments made in the Beijing Conference in 1995 was to formulate a national policy which would guide the programme and action for empowerment of women. Hence the year 2001 had been declared as the year of women's empowerment in India. The National Policy of the Empowerment of Women (NPEW) which was adopted by the government of India on 20 March 2001 is a welcome step in the right direction. The implementation of NPEW opens up large-scale opportunities for women to participate in the political, economic and social processes of the country, thereby visualising their advancement, development and empowerment. The NPEW is therefore seen as a comprehensive policy statement in the right direction and also captures the issues and concerns of the women's movement in India.

The salient features of NPEW are as follows:

- Enabling women to realize their full potential through political, economic and social policies.

- Equal access to women in power sharing and decision-making of social/political and economic life of the nation.
- Mainstreaming of gender perspective in the development process.
- Improving the legal and judicial system in India in favour of women.
- Changing societal attitudes and community practices by active participation and involvement of both men and women.
- Economic empowerment of women through measures such as easy access to credit, including women's perspectives in designing and implementing macro-economic and social policies.
- Social empowerment of women through focus on improving the system of education, health, nutrition, drinking water, housing, environment, science and technology.
- Helping women in difficult circumstances like poverty, destitution and to fight against all forms of violence faced by women.
- To ensure rights of the girl child through strict enforcement of laws against parental sex-selection, female-foeticide, female infanticide, child marriage, child abuse, etc.
- To encourage media to develop codes of conduct, guidelines and other self-regulatory mechanisms to remove gender stereotypes and promote balanced portrayals of women and men.

Recognizing the critical role that educational institutions can play in promoting social awareness regarding gender issues and also in formulation, implementation, monitoring and review of policies and programmes affecting women, the Department of Women and Child Development, Government of India provided financial assistance to Jamia Millia Islamia to focus on policy prescriptions within NPEW. As a result a regional-level two-day seminar on National Policy on the Empowerment of Women was held on the 7th and 8th March,

2002. Two organizations whose combined efforts fructified into holding the seminar were Sarojini Naidu Centre for Women's Studies and the Department of Social Work, Jamia Millia Islamia. The programme was held in various session covering aspects such as National Policy on Empowerment of women. Government and NGOs perspective socio-economic empowerment of women, political empowerment of women, minority women, with intervention for each session being made by well-known people from the field. The speakers were drawn from the world of academia and practice who made significant contributions to enliven and enrich the proceedings.

PROCEEDINGS

Inaugural Session

The inaugural session began with a welcome address by Professor A.S. Kohli, Head, Department of Social Work, Jamia Millia Islamia who spoke of the significance of the seminar and highlighted the role of universities in providing a forum for discussion of policy matters in an impartial manner. He welcomed the participants, in particular Professor Veena Majumdar, Professor Susheela Kaushik and Vice-Chancellor of Jamia Millia Islamia, Mr. Syed Shahid Mahdi. He hoped that the seminar would result in better understanding of the policy and its implementation.

Professor (Mrs.) Anjali Gandhi, the co-ordinator of the seminar spoke of the relevance of the seminar and the significance of partnership of the collaborating agencies, namely, Sarojini Naidu Centre for Women's Studies and the Department of Social Work, Jamia Millia Islamia. She highlighted, among other things, the need for a greater discussion on the policy in the light of the presence of certain lacunae, such as the absence of a media policy, the Panchayati Raj Institutions getting only a passing reference and the absence of a clear plan of action. She then briefly acquainted the participants with the outlines of the seminar.

Inaugural Address

Professor Susheela Kaushik, Director, Centre for Development Studies and Action giving the inaugural address commended the policy which had come after a long struggle for the need of such a policy as was agreed in the Beijing Conference. She regretted that the policy took six years to be formulated and yet has failed to fulfil the expectations that it had raised. The document is not being disseminated appropriately. She said that she was looking forward to seeing the action plan to implement the policy.

Professor Kaushik felt that the status of women has not improved despite the strong social reform, nationalist movements and various social legislations. In fact, the special privileges and provisions tend to make women mere dependents. Real power and development can reach women only when women emerge politically empowered and can formulate policy. Among other things, she wanted the extension of reservation policy for women in Panchayats and Nagar Palikas to State Assemblies and Parliament. This should not be seen as an end but a means to get a rightful space in the political arena. She also looked at various factors hindering empowerment, such as patriarchal apparatuses such as religion, caste, customs, economic and social backwardness, the nature of the state and its demands, steadily declining cultural standards and moral values, etc.

She felt that empowerment is to be seen as a long and continuous process. The goals of women's empowerment are also constantly changing, which poses continual challenges to both women and men. She urged that such a process should be a participatory one.

In her keynote address, Professor Veena Majumdar, President, Centre for Women's Development Studies (CWDS), New Delhi congratulated the convenors for the selection of the theme for the seminar. She, however, expressed her dissent to the formulation of a women's policy as not being able to meet the challenge of the 21st century. She pointed out that in the seventies the Committee on the Status of Women in India had recommended certain major policy changes, which have still not been implemented. Times have changed since then, bringing up with them the necessity of making drastic changes. However, the policy seems to keep looking back to the past instead of dealing with the dynamics of the present. She also questioned the legitimacy of the policy in the light of its not being deliberated by both houses of Parliament. In that sense it remains a document formulated by the civil servants of the Department of Women and Child Development and does not have the stamp of authority of people through their representatives.

She also felt that certain policy and programmatic interventions have not been evaluated and such evaluations have not been woven into the making of the policy. She regretted that there are no indications of the kind of results obtained from earlier interventions in the areas of women. She felt that such contradictions are many, which needed to be addressed by any policy document which claimed to be 'comprehensive'.

Professor Majumdar spoke of the need to understand Indian women's lives as influenced by individual, familial, regional, linguistic, cultural, occupational, class, caste, community, religion and ethical considerations and the need to broaden political identities and beliefs. Speaking of the Indian report on Gender and Governance published by CWDS she drew attention to its major insights. The whole sector of development, economic, social, education, health, political, institutional, is caught up in the dynamics of so-called reform. The State is withdrawing from the leadership and protective roles with regard to the underprivileged. There is a slow and steady erosion of the entire ideology underlying the Constitution or the struggle of the Indian people and its steady replacement with supremacy of the market. In the end, she desired women's studies to play the role of a catalyst with a reformist role. Women's studies also need to remain within existing educational institutions and indigenise social sciences.

Mr. Syed Shahid Mahdi, the then Vice Chancellor, Jamia Millia Islamia delivering the Chairperson's remarks, reflected on Professor Majumdar's unhappiness over the usages of certain clichés promoted by UN bodies but also felt that that the importance of UN bodies cannot be undermined.

He felt that the seminar was trying to give voice to the people who are working at the grassroots. He urged that empowerment of women need not be seen as affirmative action alone but has to be intensified by the entire society. The Chairperson felt that what is available in terms of policy has to be constructively and best implemented. For a beginning, one could bring out a Status Report on Women every year or two. The crucial aspects are to ensure that it is a non-official report and that the data should be disaggregated according to the different categories of women. Such an attempt would largely fulfil the need for a public monitoring system, whose critical absence has led to the limited improvement in the situation of women in spite of a plethora of policies and programmes. Speaking about Jamia Millia Islamia, he felt that the issue of women's empowerment is a vast one and requires co-ordination between the Department of Social Work, Sarojini Naidu Centre and other departments such as Mass Communication Research Centre and the Department of Fine Arts.

The Inaugural session concluded with a vote of thanks by Professor Hajira Kumar, Director, Sarojini Naidu Centre who thanked the participants for their presence. She also thanked Professor Susheela Kaushik and Veena Majumdar for their enlightening and thought-provoking ideas with regard to women's empowerment and the critical issues facing the policy.

Session II

The second session scheduled for the day was to provide an understanding of the National Policy for Empowerment of Women.

Professor P.K. Gandhi of the Department of Social Work, JMI chaired the session. Ms. Shalini Prasad, Deputy Director, DPEP in the Ministry of Human Resource Development, New Delhi was the first speaker. She focused on certain key areas for action in the educational field initiated by the government such as : equal access to education, special measures to eliminate discrimination, universalisation of education, eradication of illiteracy, creating gender-sensitive education and enhancement of the quality of education to facilitate life-long earning and develop vocational and technical skills to provide for a curriculum which is gender sensitive. In particular she provided details of the programme of action (POA, 1992) and demonstrated how the *Mahila Samakhya Programme* of the Government of India was instrumental in women's empowerment through education.

Dr. Ranjana Kumari, President, Centre for Social Research, New Delhi, giving an NGO perspective on the NPEW, felt that a policy by its very nature has to be a comprehensive one, taking into account every aspect of women's life. She pointed out that the implementing agency for the policy is none other than the body politic which has no representation by women. She also expressed her doubts about implementation of the policy in the absence of a gender-just budget where less than 0.87% of the resources go to women-related programmes. She also cited the case of micro credit pointing out that it received only 2% of the funds available with banking systems. She expressed doubts on how such a policy could then be implemented. She emphasized that the delivery system has no resources for implementing the policy and that there is a marked absence of women in decision-making. She posited this in the context of a failed promise of 33% of resources from all ministries' budgets to be spent on gender-related activities. She expressed her doubts about the sincerity of intended action by citing the pending Bills in parliament related to domestic violence and women's reservation. She also lamented the absence of a proper monitoring mechanism for policy implementation.

Intervening in the debate Mr. Yashpal Dabas, Under Secretary in the HRD Ministry, informed that for the monitoring of policy a National Council at the Central level has been formed which is located within the Prime Ministers' office (PMO) and there is a state-level monitoring by the Chief Minister's secretariat.

When the discussion was opened for wider participation,

Professor Kaushik felt that the NPEW seems to be an aggregation of all the policies put together. However, it lacked vision and did not seem to reflect the aspirations of women.

The discussion further focused on the lack of clarity in the definition of the term empowerment, and lack of an action plan on policy implementation. It was suggested that the action plan must be made drawing from grassroot experiences as well as the onus of implementation should be at the district level but not centralised within DM's office and that it should reach the last woman. The general feeling of the participants was that a more comprehensive effort of policy formulation has to be undertaken afresh, weaving in various perspectives and speaking with a clear focus.

Session III

The session on socio-economic empowerment was chaired by Dr. Anil Kalia, Director, Child Survival India, New Delhi who intervening as a resource person, also focused on various aspects in the area. Professor Ratna Verma, Department of Social Work, Delhi University focused on woman as an individual, a member of the family and society and explored the various factors hampering her empowerment.

Professor Tulsi Patel, Department of Sociology, Delhi School of Economics, University of Delhi, speaking in the context of woman's individuality, explored her predicament in the social situation which curtails her individual freedom. She historically traced women's exclusion in matters of governance, rights and citizenship. She felt that it is important to understand how we look at women when we study socio-economic empowerment. The identity of woman is entirely focused on her body as a reproductive unit, and fertility and motherhood are key terms in understanding women. Women do not have control over their bodies. This control lies with 'men', 'state' and institutions of religion which are powerful. The idea of equality and the idea of individuality of women is not present in the policy on empowerment. Though legally, women seem to enjoy equal rights, they are not equal in the society and at home. The emerging concern of female foeticide leading to the decline of sex ratio, specially between 0 and 6 years in states like Gujarat, Haryana, and Maharashtra does not find a place in the policy. The need for rethinking the patriarchal society which places a stumbling block in women's empowerment has to be addressed both at policy and programmatic level.

Dr. Promila Kapur, Director, Integrated Human Development Services Foundation, New Delhi and a woman writer, expressed her concern regarding the low status of women in society. She attributed this to differential socialization of girls and boys. She focused on the oppressive traditions, customs, ideologies, social institutions and inherent inequities in the social structure which pose difficulty in the family. She lamented that there is a lack of trust and caring relationships within the family. She felt that there is large-scale infiltration of negative values within the family set up, leading to violence against women. Added to this is the already existing unhealthy gender-biased values and attitudes of men, women and the society at large towards the girl child and women. There is a need, she felt, to strengthen marital and family relationship and family life education. She felt that the policy should focus on women within the family and their socio-economic empowerment.

Dr. Zarina Bhatty, President, Indian Association for Women Studies spoke about the situation of women in India. The considerable statistical presence of women at work and absence in other areas is reflected in the fact that women work 3085 hours in a year. Of the executive positions in India, only 6% women are represented in Indian Parliament and 4% in State Legislatures. Women hold only 1% of the property in India. Most of the domestic work is not valued as work. Ninety per cent of working women are from the unorganised sector. Women constitute 70% of the poor in India. In spite of such a large presence in terms of needs, Dr. Bhatty felt that development planners perceive women only as a means for reproduction and not as a resource-generating mechanism. She also felt that institutional mechanisms are inadequate for arresting the exploitation of women or in perpetuating the status of women. She regretted that 85% of the registered gynaecologists indulged in sex-determination tests in Mumbai. While appreciating the National Policy on Empowerment of Women, Dr. Bhatty pointed out that there was no specific allocation of funds and accountability in the policy and that it was silent on the mental health of women though it speaks on women's health issues. She felt that issues that needed attention were in the areas of accountability of the concerned institutions, lack of resources, and the need to change the mind-set of both men and women. In this connection she felt that universities and women's studies centres should be watchdogs.

Ms. Maitree Chaudhary, Associate Professor, Centre for Study of Social System, School of Social Sciences, Jawaharlal Nehru University, New Delhi identified the following constrictive elements in women's empowerment: the family based on patriarchy, which discriminates among male and female; the caste communities as well as religious sects which discriminate and uphold the lower status of women; and the state with its political system which has an ideology that does not favour women. In addition, the globalisation process exploits women. There is commodification of women and marketisation throughout the world with mass competition that ensures that women are marginalized. She felt that the policy should focus on retrieving a place for women and rescuing them from their marginalized status. In this she called for a free look at the 1938 document of the Karachi Congress which gave equal position to women and observed that it should once again be recalled for shaping the policy. She emphasized that choices and decisions needed to be made collectively and these should have a place in policy.

Dr. S.L. Manga from 'Santulan' said that the policy is lacking in any notion of mental health. The policy should reflect on changing the mind-sets that create discrimination between men and women. From the point of intervention, two broad factors in psycho-social problems could be identified. One is located in bio-genics, which involves bio-chemistry and necessarily demands medical intervention, and the second is located in family and the environment. Hence a change in the environment, a change in the behaviour of the 'significant' others is also required. The intervention should focus on valuing all women as having the potential to empower themselves.

Professor Paul Sachdev of Memorial University, Canada spoke on the elusiveness of the notion of equality. For him empowerment requires assertiveness as against aggressiveness. The status of woman in health-related issues is a reflection of her status in society. Especially concerning HIV/AIDS issues, women are vulnerable both because of their traditional submissive role and inability to exercise their rights. Commercialisation of women's bodies is a major issue and there is a need for women to fight to exercise their rights by negotiation rather than by resorting to violence. He felt that not only economic but other socio-cultural factors needed to be addressed for improving the status of women and focus on HIV/AIDS requires focus on protected sex with a need to make available female condoms.

Dr. Anil Kalia, Director, Child Survival India, looking at the status of women in India felt that women's vulnerability is due to age-old customs and traditions. Woman is a victim in the family, society and market. There is a need for looking at change and defining it appropriately as well as focusing on the grassroots where minimum facilities are lacking. The policy should reflect on the tangible things that women need right now, which also calls for defining such needs.

Political Empowerment

The session on political empowerment was chaired by Professor M.Z. Khan, Department of Social Work, JMI. The Resource Person was Professor Rajeshwar Prasad, Former Director, Institute of Social Sciences, New Delhi.

Ms. Kiran Wadhera, President, Asian Centre of Organization, Research and Development (ACORD), speaking on political empowerment through local self-government, felt that traditions and cultural practices still dominate society and are the main contributing factors towards exploitation of women. In this regard she felt that NGOs' intervention is needed to improve the condition of women. According to her, only those who have a say in the decision making process are empowered.

Dr. A.S. Narang, Professor, Indira Gandhi National Open University speaking on the process of empowerment through legislation felt that there is lack of justice and empowerment due to the existing mind-sets, conventions, traditions, religious and cultural values and their interpretation. On the other hand, implementation mechanisms are inadequate or non-existent. He felt that there is a need for sensitization of the judiciary for implementing the law.

Ms. Urvashi Butalia, writer and pioneer of Women's Press, spoke about women's empowerment becoming everybody's responsibility rather than the state's responsibility alone. She felt that even though laws exist, few benefit women. The decisions made at the level of judiciary often undermine women's rights and the existing infrastructure denies full exercise of women's rights. There is a need to critically look at law and policies, she asserted. She also felt that policy formulation should have been participatory.

Dr. A.N. Singh, Professor, University of Kurukshetra spoke on the 73rd Amendment of the Constitution and the problems of empowerment. He expressed his happiness that the 73rd Amendment has given a platform for women to look after their problems. He enlightened the audience regarding a study made on participation of Scheduled Caste women in decision-making and shared its recommendations. He suggested that there is a need for training and education for women, specially those belonging to the scheduled caste. Family support is needed, he felt, so that they can function effectively in the Panchayat. He also felt that there is a need for controlling the restrictive effects of society.

Professor Rajeshwar Prasad, founder member Indian Social Science Association intervening as the resource person, spoke of the importance of power sharing in a democratic society. He said that there is a need for emancipation of women from tradition and constraints imposed by religion. Tradition must be understood and changed if necessary and rejected if found unfavourable to gender justice. Such an emancipation, he said, is a must for economic empowerment and ownership of means of production. The process of emancipation at the social, political and cultural level cannot be done by legislation alone and requires concerted effort by one and all.

Professor M.Z. Khan, Chairperson of the session, remarked that there is a need for increasing participation of women in all spheres with lessening of control by family and community on the life of a woman. Women's empowerment should not mean destruction of interpersonal relations but it should help in restoring balance within the family. The disciplines of social work and sociology must concentrate on the importance of women's political participation, so that they can function effectively in the panchayat. He also felt that there is a need for re-structuring the social system.

Minority Women : Issues and Empowerment

The session on minority women was chaired by Professor Mohini Anjum of the Department of Sociology, JMI. The resource person was Mr. Tahir Mahmood, Former Chairman, Minority Commission of India, who requested everyone concerned not to compartmentalize women into minority/ majority sections. In this regard he felt that any gender differences emerging from within laws needed to be addressed as well as efforts should be made towards uniformity and not segregation by asking for separate laws for each section of society.

Professor Siddiqui, Department of Social Work, JMI began with the role of education in empowerment of women and felt that this is a crucial component in the process of empowerment. A fundamental change was required in the male psyche wherein lies the root of gender inequality.

Mr. Anees Ahmad a practising lawyer felt that the Constitution gave equal rights to men and women, however, there need to be special provisions so that an unequal partner be placed at par with equal partner. He felt that biases and prejudices towards personal law as far as Muslim women are concerned came forth in the interpretation of secular laws. According to him, institutions of civil society and the Constitution have failed to fulfil the expectations of the people, particularly women.

There is a need for having gender-just laws for the whole of the country as personal laws deny protection to women. He also felt that secular laws are no better in providing justice to women with relation to the institution of marriage, hence there was a need for amending them suitably.

Mr. Y.S. Alone, Lecturer, Department of Fine Arts, Kurukshetra University, spoke on the status of Buddhist women. He felt that there is a need to understand the position of marginalized women not just from a framework of economic deprivation but also broadly from the concern of social inequality based on religion and cultural practice of Indian society. Buddhist women also are to be seen juxtaposed between their lower status within their own community as well as the attitude from the hegemonic tradition of the larger society. In addition women have to face large-scale discrimination and denial of equal opportunities. Another concern is that there is no legal recognition of the Buddhist marriage system. In this scenario one should have a re-look at caste-based gender discrimination for understanding minority women. There is a need for changing mind-set and laws to make it possible for minority women to exercise their rights. The policy then can begin by first focusing on minority women, which the present National Policy fails to recognise. There is a need to allocate resources to several social categories separately and also involving women in the making of personal laws for minority women.

Manisha Sethi, Assistant Editor Biblio: a Review of Books spoke on issues covering Jain Women. She pointed out that in the Indian Constitution, Jain is included under the rubric of 'Hindu' as part of Article 25. She then explored the status of women and felt that in spite of favourable social statistics as per the sex ratio (946/1000) as also of comparable literacy levels between men and women, there are problems that Jain women face. Specially focusing on the religious and philosophical positions of Jainism, she spoke of a son preference and gendered division of religious duties as a major hindrance to equality of Jain women within their community. There is an influence of patriarchal culture in Jainism, hence the status of Jain women is lower. She also mentioned that Jain women do not hold economic power within their community. The status and position of Jain women thus would be understood only by locating them within patriarchal structures. The essentially patriarchal nature of religious practice tones down the notion of equality prevalent philosophy positions. She felt that hardly any forum exists to change the position. Understanding of divergence of State ideals of womanhood and the position of women that exists in reality is crucial to understand the minority status of Jain women within their society.

Margaret Antony of Indian Social Institute, New Delhi speaking on Christian women noted that Christians constitute 2.5% of the Indian population, of which 75% are tribal groups. There are biases against women within the Christian religion which she explored at length. She regretted that in spite of promise of a better life through conversions, the plight of Dalit Christian women is vulnerable because of caste, class and gender inequalities. She articulated the concerns of Christian women and pointed out that there is alienation of Dalit Christian women within their community and also outside. This alienation is also reflected in their personal laws in matters of right to divorce and separation and the functioning of such laws within the patriarchal paradigm. She expressed the hope that such issues find a place in the policy.

Valedictory Session

Ms. Razia Ismail, ex-President, World Young Women's Christian Association (YWCA) and President, Women's Coalition, New Delhi delivered the valedictory address. She emphasized the need for assessing a woman's worth and the idea of her empowerment on the measure of human worth not limited to motherhood. Women are not a category, she said. They are citizens with as much rights and privileges as anyone. She felt that the National Policy for Empowerment for Women fails to recognise women as persons and citizens and merely looks at them as another category which needs empowerment. She felt that any policy which commits such a mistake by its very nature becomes self-limiting. She demanded that woman be seen much beyond her reproductive functions and that she be recognized for her worth in productive activities.

Ms Ismail felt that instead of looking at women as victims and as beneficiaries in need of many services, one should look at them as equal, participating citizens. The whole perspective needs to have a change so that one recognises people, citizens and human beings acknowledging their worth and potential and at the same time daring to recognise that about half of these people are female. She felt that one must move beyond sub typing people as female and male as all are humans and human resources. She insisted that both policy and programmes relating to women should be positioned in the conceptual framework of human rights and of citizens' role in society and nation.

Ms Ismail felt that the National Policy on Empowerment of Women imposes on people the limited identity of being a 'woman' as the defining identity. She questioned the intent of 'women friendliness' in the policies positioned in the context of studies which speak of gender-unjust budgets. Ms Ismail felt that the female's personhood and citizenship are above gender. One may have any number of identities and one of them could be female. This she felt could be used to position one's consideration of gender and gender justice and therefore can be used to assess the policy.

Critically examining the policy, Ms Ismail questioned the rationale of such women-specific intervention as providing for 100 women scientists as part of Science and Technology Policy. She expressed her doubts that intentions of welfare reflected in the policy hardly cater to the needs of gender justice and help female Indians to take their rightful place as people.

Ms Ismail felt that instead of treating people as categories to be provided for under various welfare schemes ostensibly to provide justice, the existing policies, laws and commissions should look at one human development policy and vision, which would cover all people in India. She desired that the citizens of India should take the opportunity to frame and draft a National Policy for Human Rights as an approach to human resource development.

She urged for gender profiling of child development and child rights and linking of agendas that affect people. She felt that the state should not be absolved of its responsibility to do this and answer for it specially in the light of the lack of commitment to financing and managing minimum essential improvements in survival, health, nutrition, education, shelter, social and legal protection.

Dr. Jyoti Kakkar presented a Summary of the proceedings of the Seminar.

The Chairperson of the valedictory session was Professor Surendra Singh, President, Association of School of Social Work in India and Head, Department of Social Work, Lucknow University. He felt that there is a lot that can be done with regard to the policy and there is a need for constant vigil about the goals, outcomes, procedures, programmes, and implementing and monitoring mechanisms.

Professor Anjali Gandhi, co-ordinator of the Seminar welcomed the participants for the valedictory session and congratulated them for their valuable contributions to the seminar.

Professor S.M. Sajid of the Department of Social Work proposed the Vote of Thanks.

Suggestions Emerging from Seminar Discussion

1. The women's policy must be backed by political will and budget allocations. The *Mahila Samakhaya Programme*, in pursuance of the National Policy of Education 1986, which evolved through the process of consultation was pointed out as one example.
2. The empowerment of women is in fact an empowerment of society and hence is a responsibility of all stake-holders who should work in tandem with each other.
3. A National Policy Status Report for Women should be

brought out annually by an independent body to give a clear indication of various dimensions of women's status.

4. Policies should reflect the aspirations of women and women's movement and be formulated keeping in mind age specific women groups.
5. Policies should be framed keeping in view the ground realities and social structure.
6. Women's policy should be formulated with a gender perspective in partnership with and participation of women especially women from the grassroots.
7. There is a need to make changes in the National Policy for women and amend it suitably for it to be applicable and effective with regard to minority women.
8. Policies should be followed by time-bound action plans.
9. There should be decentralisation of power and finances to the grassroots to ensure proper implementation of the policy.
10. There is a need for gender auditing of budgets by women's groups and or statutory bodies.
11. The policy should have definite guidelines for gender budgeting and also for monitoring the actual expenditure pattern to ensure that the engendered budget gets implemented.
12. The population policies which are punitive in nature and act as a disincentive for women empowerment should be reviewed.
13. There should be a single family law for women from all communities. There is a need for codification of traditional laws and customs, so that arbitrary, gender-sensitive practices can be checked.
14. There is a need for review of customary laws that are discriminatory towards women, like those on property and inheritance.
15. Education should be made gender-sensitive from the primary level so that boys and girls are sensitized to problems like gender inequality, child abuse, child marriage, dowry system, etc.

16. There is a need for sensitizing men and including them in all women's empowerment programmes.
17. There is a need for sensitization of the print and audio-visual media towards women's empowerment.
18. Women's study centres at the Universities should be strengthened so that they can play a constructive role in the issue of women's empowerment.
19. There is a need for adequate literature on subjects related to women which among others include minority women, women and health, gender budgeting, etc.

The participants of the seminar identified the strengths of the National Policy for Empowerment of Women as follows :-

a. It is an effort to place a coordinated policy for women in one place.
b. It proposes the formation of a national apex body.

The weaknesses of the **National Policy** pointed out were as follows:

1. The policy has been formulated without a dialogue with the stakeholders. It has not been debated or discussed.
2. Many of the recommendations made by the NGOs have not been incorporated.
3. The document lacks a clear-cut vision, structure, framework and plan of action. In fact, it is only a collection of existing policies.
4. Special strategies for participation of women in the political process as a result of the 73rd and 74th Amendments had not been thought of.
5. The reservation of women in the Parliament has been incorporated in the political scenario but no special provisions have been made to tackle the situation.

Index